MW00471946

From 10 To 5

My Journey With Diabetes

Ahmed Afifi

Copyright © 2019 Ahmed Afifi
All rights reserved.
ISBN: 9781794649583

Disclaimer

This publication contains information that is intended to help the readers be better-informed consumers of health care. It is presented as general advice on health care. It is not intended to be a substitute for the medical advice of a licensed physician. The publisher and author are not engaged in rendering medical or other professional services. Always consult your doctor for your individual needs.

To my Wife Rehab, for the endless support, for the unconditional love, and for the hypo nights. Your fingerprints are all over my diabetes journey.

If insulin is my life, you are my insulin.

To my precious children Habiba, Omar and Salma.

To all People with diabetes with love and sincere wishes with controlled blood sugar.

Table of Contents

Acknowledgement

Managing diabetes is a nightmare without a loving and caring partner. Writing a book in diabetes management is not an easy mission. I wasn't able to either control my diabetes or write this book without the tremendous support I received from Rehab, my lovely wife. She granted me the gift of her time to go through every line of this book by relentlessly reading the early drafts tens of times. She directed me to many shortcomings and guided me to write a book with a beautiful soul, just like her. It is only because of her this book became reality.

Special thanks to you, my friend Carole friend for the great support you extended to me in reviewing and editing this book. Thanks for the great foreword you wrote and for the excellent chapter you honored this book with. I am so grateful to you Carole for your editorial help, your precious time, technical diabetes expertise, caring insight, and valuable friendship.

Special thanks to Dr. Gary Fettke for being kind and humble enough to honor me with such an insightful foreword of this book. The foreword reveals an authentic character of a real scientist and a noble human being. Dr. Gary, you are a hero, an icon for bravery and I am extremely proud of knowing you.

Ahmed Afifi

__Foreword__

In my naivety some years ago, I had no idea of my own journey when I was encouraged by my wife and daughter to embrace Facebook, Twitter, YouTube and the like with my 'No Fructose' message, which has evolved into a 'Low Carb Healthy Fat' lifestyle for myself and others.

I certainly had no idea of the number of individuals I have had the opportunity and honor to support by openly stating that I, as a doctor, got it wrong for so many years when it came to the understanding and management of diabetes in all of its forms.

I was not taught, and it is still not, that diabetes is essentially an inability of the body to manage the glucose load that it is presented with. Reduce the load and the complications are completely avoidable. Reduce the insulin load and the yo-yo existence of poor blood glucose control and health outcomes effectively vanish overnight.

A few years ago, I met Ahmed Afifi via the amazing social media world we live in. I had no understanding that I was part of his journey and his request for me to write a foreword to his writings humbles me.

Ahmed is not a doctor nor a health professional. He is an engineer and is one of several engineers that I know in the Low Carb world that understand the issues surrounding diabetes and blood glucose control better than most doctors. They have their own journeys of themselves or their loved ones. Once they see the simplicity of the numbers, there is an overwhelming desire to share the message for the sake of others. There is a purpose for improving, that we all share.

There is also anger and frustration towards the medical profession for not embracing this concept. That emotion is well founded as 'guidelines' in the management of diabetes have been shaped by vested interests for the last several decades. Challenging those guidelines that have become rulebooks comes at a price for patients as well as doctors. The Internet and Social Media is giving a voice to those questioning the paradigm.

As a surgeon, my life is based around my surgical skills but as time has progressed, I realize that my teachings are having a further reach. *'The pen is truly mightier than the sword'* or it could be rewritten in today's terms as the *'Tweet has a greater reach than the scalpel'*.

Ahmed's first foray into writing was in Arabic as there was and remains a dearth of current literature for his community. He is making a difference. "From Ten to Five" sounds like a measurement of time and in a way it is. Ahmed's improvement in his diabetes control is literally buying him time.

"From Ten to Five" is not a prescription on how to manage diabetes exactly. It is an introduction to the concepts of lowering carbohydrate intake, managing protein and healthy fat content, an overall vision about insulin relationship with obesity, emphasizing of the importance of achieving normal blood sugar and considering the options around drug management and particularly medication reduction.

This books' great strength lies in the individual stories wound into the body of information. I truly was moved when reading the personal aspects of how diabetes affects the individual, and particularly in poorer and less educated communities. The inability to access sound medical advice, let alone appropriate medication, is an enormous problem. Western medicine does not have that sorted out either, but the problems are amplified in the stories Ahmed tells.

The issues are not just about health but cultural as well. They are personal, professional, and relearning needs to be done by health professionals and the community. Two of the stories reflected humility beautifully.

The ability to admit one's mistakes truly sets you free. That has been my journey and Ahmed's "From Ten to Five" message is going to set others free.

Gary Fettke.
M.B.,B.S.,F.R.A.C.S.(Ortho), F.A.Orth.A.
Orthopedic Surgeon and Low Carbohydrates Healthy Fat (LCHF) advocate.
Tasmania, Australia.

Second foreword

Ahmed Afifi is not a medical professional. So, why read his book about diabetes? Ahmed is one of us. Diabetes is as real to him as it is to you. I know diabetes is real to you or someone you love dearly or you would not be reading these words. I know, too, that you are struggling with diabetes or you would not need this book. In these pages, Ahmed shows you his challenges. He shares his experience, his research, and his spirit so that your journey to normal blood sugar may be shorter and lighter.

Ahmed's first book published in Arabic and his social media outlets have reached over 26,000 people in parts of the world foreign to us. He now delivers to us in English, the disparity of information and resources for people suffering from diabetes all over the world. We witness his passion to shed light not only on this injustice but also on the tragedy of misinformation on diabetes management for the rich and the poor alike.

While I have never met Ahmed in person, I have held him in great esteem for his advocacy ever since we met through social media. As I read this unique mixture of memoir and diabetes education, I realized that despite being separated by a hemisphere;

we had been on the same path at the same time. Ahmed was learning things for his health and I, for my then five-year-old daughter who had been diagnosed with Type 1 diabetes nearly 3 years prior. Despite differences in geography, language, culture, gender, profession and nearly any other demographic, you can think of, we have found a shared neurological circuitry.

Achieving near-normal blood sugar after struggling for years to earnestly follow mainstream recommendations leaves an indelible mark on your soul that is never erased. Our shared synapses have made it a great pleasure to help him clarify his voice in a second language. I have been honored to be invited on just a few steps of the long journey that led to this inspiring work.

With this book in your hands, travel swiftly and may the road rise up to meet you.

Carole Friend.

Introduction

I can still feel the overwhelming frustration from when I was first diagnosed with diabetes back in 2003. At that time, the information about real control of blood sugar was scarce. Physicians have almost no time to spend with People with diabetes (PWD) to explain the major concepts of diabetes control. Concepts like; what to eat, when to eat, insulin factors, how and where to inject insulin, why they must use this type of insulin instead of another and much more crucial information. The culture of low carbohydrate (LC) way of eating (WOE) was not well known yet. Pinpointing a doctor who tells you that bread raises your blood sugar so rapidly and massively was like seeing a polar bear in Sahara desert. Finding myself in the dilemma of having uncontrolled diabetes despite following the physician's instructions word for word, filled my soul with sadness and despair. I felt lost and dispersed.

I am not a physician or a nutritionist. I am a mechanical engineer, and, now an Associate Diabetes Educator. Prior to that, I was an insulin-dependent diabetic struggling with uncontrolled diabetes. With the grace of God and by reading, learning, searching and applying all to myself, I was capable to go from being way out of control to excellent control beyond my wildest imagination: from an HbA1c of 10 to HbA1c of 5.5.

My ultimate goal in writing this book is to share with you my own experience. I want to show you how I was able to control my blood sugar and the long process that allowed me to avoid the never-ending cycle of hyperglycemia and hypoglycemia. I want you to understand how changing the way I ate enabled me to have such a dramatic improvement. I want to prove to you how keeping your weight in check could improve your insulin sensitivity. Imagine an HbA1c of 10 and over to an HbA1c of 5.5 seemingly overnight! I am not suggesting that this is the right approach for everyone. I am not also suggesting that it is the sole method to achieve such tight control. On the contrary, I am quite aware we are all different. Instead, I emphasize that despite our differences, there are common factors that have a similar positive influence on our different versions of diabetes.

Knowledge is power. On my journey, I have learned many things mainstream medicine never taught me. These were the missing pieces I needed. Many changes in our daily lives dealing with diabetes will reward us greatly in our struggle to achieve normal blood sugar: food choices, multiple daily injection (MDI) techniques, matching food with insulin, daily exercise, getting the needed support from your partner, prolonged and intermittent fasting. I want you to have the benefit of my journey so that your path will be smoother. This is my gift to you. Take what works for you and leave the rest.

When I started to spread the knowledge about diabetes management through my FB page, my first book <u>What You Do Not Know About Diabetes</u>, written in Arabic, other FB diabetes groups and through my website, I was saddened by the magnitude of the confusion among people with diabetes in the Middle East and, indeed, all over the world. Their frustration of continuous and severe blood sugar fluctuation astonished me. I realized that the majority of people with diabetes are not able to find the right information needed to guide them to good blood sugar control. I understood their confusion because I had walked the same path.

It may surprise you that I am shedding light on major concepts, not minor ones. You will read some real-life stories, which offer insight into the real importance of controlling diabetes. I will address subjects that might seem a bit far from diabetes but have a real and meaningful impact on diabetes control. I will discuss food choices, obesity, dietary habits, insulin resistance, leptin resistance, cholesterol, the role of insulin, weight control, low carb way of eating and, most importantly, my journey to get from HbA1c of 10 to HbA1c of 5.5. You will find me instructively criticizing the mainstreamers, the physicians who care more about the guidelines of big organizations and governmental institutions and do not see the drawbacks and the poor results inflicting harsh complications on PWD who follow those guidelines day in and day out. In the meantime, I tip my hat for those knowledgeable physicians, nutritionists, and scientists who seek the truth.

I will use simple language and not a complicated medical one. I will just recount my story and share any experience that helped me to normalize my blood sugar. In fact, I figured out that my story is the story of many who walked the same path but with different details.

It is my humble wish that my experience will open the eyes of people with diabetes that control is within their reach. I believe this book is not only for people with diabetes but it is for health seekers, pre-diabetics, people who want to lose weight and fasting lovers. I put this book in your hands to give you hope that you too can control your blood sugar and live a good life. Additionally, I hope my message can make it possible for pre-diabetics and non-diabetics to keep the diabetes ghost at bay.
Hope you like the book.

Ahmed Afifi.

Chapter 1: It was never easy

"Of course, there was a lot of anger and denial and even attempts to forget about being diabetic. Maybe I could forget about it for a while, but it never forgot about me."

Dr. Richard K. Bernstein

In 2003, by the age of 35, I found out, the hard way, I had T2 diabetes after experiencing the familiar symptoms, such as endless thirst, frequent urination, exhaustion, and endless hunger. At the time, I did not realize what was actually taking place, as I was clueless about diabetes. I visited my physician, assuming there was nothing serious to worry about. Overwhelmingly, my random blood sugar test was 460 mg/dl along with HbA1c of 12. Just like that, in one minute, I entered the diabetes club and rotated in its vicious circle.

A few years before this diagnosis, I passed through metabolic syndrome stages without realizing it. It all started with gradual weight gain around my midsection in four years. At the same time, I had a huge rise in my Triglyceride (TG) numbers along with craving fast-acting carbohydrates (FAC) like sugar, bread, pasta, juices, fruits, and, rice. In those four years, I gained around a horrible 70 pounds.

The pattern of gaining weight, high triglyceride, and slightly elevated blood pressure is a common pattern we can notice all around us nowadays. This pattern takes years to build up. Unfortunately, in my case, it went by unnoticed until it led to insulin resistance, metabolic syndrome and then diabetes. At that time, our medical knowledge used to be received directly from our physicians. The internet was not common yet. There was no chance to learn more about your illness if you want to.

Initially, it was difficult to deal with diabetes, both physically and emotionally. I had a continuous high blood sugar numbers interrupted by multiple episodes of hypoglycemia. This pattern left me feeling battered at the end of every day. My blood sugar profile was terrible despite carefully following the advice given by endos, diabetes educators and nutritionists. Sadly, they think they are giving us the right advice. Yet, nothing could be further from the truth, as I learned later.

In fact, their advice was (and still is) based on major diabetes organizations' guidelines. Unfortunately, those guidelines hindered any possibility of achieving normal blood sugar for me and for many people with diabetes all over the world. Let me give some examples of these misleading advice that I followed many years:

- Whole wheat and all browns (brown rice, brown pasta, and brown bread) are friends of people with diabetes.
- Five to six servings per day of fruits and vegetables are necessary.
- Eat every three to four hours.
- It is acceptable and even expected that your blood sugar may reach as high as 180 mg/dl after meals.
- HbA1c of seven or below is your target, but seven is acceptable.

- Avoid eating fat by any means because it is bad to your diabetes and to your health in general.
- Later on, when your diabetes remains uncontrolled, use fixed doses of fast-acting insulin (FAI) or pre-mixed insulin.
- Don't deprive yourself of food. There is no need to avoid eating fast-acting carbohydrates. You can eat whatever you want and inject insulin / take your pills accordingly.
- Mild hyperglycemia is acceptable in order to avoid hypoglycemia!
- Diabetes is a progressive disease even if you control it. In other words, your condition will inevitably deteriorate no matter what you do; it is a matter of time!

Additionally, my physician did not order a C-peptide lab test for me. This test measures the amount of insulin production from your beta cells (insulin-producing cells of your pancreas). Nor did he order any other special lab test for determining which type of diabetes I had. Instead, he assumed I was a T2 and immediately put me on sulfonylureas (SN) which are the current standards of care for T2. I have since found out that I have Latent Autoimmune Diabetes of Adults (LADA), which is a type of diabetes that is characterized by both decreased insulin sensitivity (like T2) and decreased insulin production (like T1).

Ironically, Sulfonylureas pushes the pancreas to produce more insulin. This causes more stress to an already stressed pancreas and finished off whatever remained of my Beta cells ability to produce insulin in about two years max.[1] Seven years later, I was astonished by what Dr. Bernstein wrote about Sulfonylureas in his book <u>Dr. Bernstein's Diabetes Solution</u>. He said, *"Most of the Oral Hypoglycemic agents (OHAs) on the market are not insulin-sensitizing or mimetic. Instead, they provoke the pancreas to produce more insulin. For several reasons, this is considerably less desirable than taking a medication that sensitizes you to insulin. First, the pancreas-provoking OHAs can cause dangerously low blood sugar levels (hypoglycemia) if used improperly or if meals are skipped or delayed. Furthermore, forcing an already overworked pancreas to produce yet more insulin can lead to the burnout of remaining beta cells. These products also facilitate beta cell destruction by increasing levels of a toxic substance called amyloid. Finally, it has been repeatedly shown in experiments—and I have seen it in my own patients—that controlling diabetes through blood sugar normalization can help restore weakened or damaged beta cells. It makes absolutely no sense to prescribe or recommend agents that will cause them renewed damage. In a nutshell, pancreas-provoking drugs are counterproductive and no longer have any place in the sensible treatment of diabetes."[2]*

He added, "Tell your doctor you do not want any product containing an agent that works by causing the pancreas to make more insulin."[3] I wished I knew this before it was too late. What Dr. Bernstein mentioned is exactly what happened to me and I hope it will not happen to you. Especially that you know now the effect of these drugs on your beta cells and your diabetes control in general.

I was riding a blood sugar rollercoaster. My blood sugar was teetering up and down severely during the twenty-four hours while my consumption of whole-wheat grains fought back and forth with my sulfonylureas.

Despite literally following the given instructions, my blood sugar results were always disappointing. Not surprisingly, I was extremely frustrated. Every time my BS goes out of control, my physician raises up my SN dose (which is a systematic protocol in dealing with T2 diabetes) until we reached the maximum dose in about three years after diagnosis. At that time, I believed my beta cells were already burned out.

Then I was prescribed Avandia, then Januvia, Actos, Janumet, Galvus met, etc. All of which had their own, insane side effects and, simultaneously, did nothing to stabilize my BS. At that point, I knew, I needed INSULIN badly. In general, my numbers were never below 200 mg/dl regardless of what medicine I took. However, many physicians, in my part of the world, are afraid to prescribe insulin to a person with diabetes. They exhaust all of their options with oral medication and press on even if the patient does not achieve good control.

They try every single pill possible until the beta cell destruction continues and insulin production is depleted. This is exactly what happened to me. Tragically, some of those who are considered T2 are, in fact, not T2. They are either LADA or Mature Onset Diabetes of the Young (MODY) which both require a different approach to treatment.

I wish I could have known then what I know now. I have since learned from Dr. Richard Bernstein that if the right low carb food and Metformin can't bring down BS, then small amounts of insulin should be used to bring the BS down in order to preserve beta cells from more depletion. **I learned that high BS creates a toxic environment that surrounds the beta cells and speeds up their destruction.**

Was it time to start injecting insulin?

To make a long story short, after five years of trying many pills, one physician started me on Lantus (Long-acting Insulin). Unquestionably, Lantus alone couldn't do much to control my BS, as I was suffering from severe glucose intolerance and needed fast-acting insulin (FAI) badly with food. However, it was hard to persuade many physicians I consulted to prescribe me FAI at the time! It is so mysterious **why most of the physicians hesitate to prescribe insulin**. Perhaps they assume most PWD hate injections or maybe they think many of them are scared of injecting insulin. Either way, I have not found this to be true for most of PWD I have met with.

Furthermore, many physicians believe it is too risky to prescribe insulin to someone who knows nothing about insulin. Physicians know how difficult and time consuming it is for them to educate their diabetic patients about the basics of diabetes control with insulin usage. They need to go deeply through issues such as insulin to carb ratio, correction factor, insulin on board, carbs counting, glycemic index and glycemic load, etc.

At the same time, many of them are not advocates of normalizing blood sugar. Apparently, they are convinced that BS numbers their patients achieve with pills are fair enough to postpone using insulin for now. Another hidden reason: they are more worried about the danger of severe hypoglycemia.

It is worth mentioning that, in our side of the world, the profession of diabetes educator rarely exists. Therefore, many physicians might think if the pills partially control blood sugar, let us stay safe instead of adding the risk of using insulin without the aid of a diabetes educator. In other words, it is easier to try all kinds of pills to the maximum extent, and suffer the consequences of less optimal control, rather than start earlier with insulin and take the risk of hypoglycemia. While in western countries, physicians are scared of being sued because of any severe hypoglycemic episode that might happen to their patients. Being in need to insulin and not able to get your physician to prescribe it for you is one of the biggest problems stops many people with diabetes from achieving normal BS.

I would also argue that many physicians are not well experienced with insulin usage. Most of them are not knowledgeable about adjusting the dosage, the timing, the factors, matching the dose with the carbohydrates count, etc. They have a weight or age charts that lead them to decide approximately the total number of daily dose of insulin for both basal and bolus and that is it! Consequently, the unfortunate person with diabetes (whom I was one of) injects steady doses of fast-acting or pre-mixed insulin two to three times a day and suffer from one of three things:

- Hypoglycemia most of the time if the dose is higher than the dose required for the meal.
- Hyperglycemia if the dose is less than required for the meal.

- Wrong timing of insulin injection could get your BS in a yoyo condition, even if the dose matches the food.

In brief, by prescribing a fixed dose of FAI, many physicians force their diabetic patients to eat continuously to cover the insulin injected, **instead of injecting the exact insulin dose needed to cover the meal. By matching the insulin dose to the meal, you can better mimic the work of pancreas.** *This is one of the first lessons, I learned, that helped me control my blood sugar.*

Why pre-Mixed insulin does not work

Back to my story, of course, Lantus alone, as basal insulin, did not do the job. So, instead of prescribing me any fast or short-acting insulin, as expected, my physician took me off Lantus and prescribed me pre-mixed insulin (30%–70%) which was one of my worst nightmares in my journey with diabetes management. Pre-mixed insulin (30-70) is a combination of short-acting insulin (30%) and intermediate-acting insulin (70%) and it comes with 50-50 as well. With pre-mixed insulin, it was impossible to control BS because, basically, when you inject such insulin, you assume the pancreas is secreting both bolus (meal insulin) and basal (background insulin) insulin in a fixed and premixed percentage of 30% – 70% respectively and that doesn't happen in reality.

In fact, if I intend to eat only healthy fat and protein with some leafy vegetables, then I will need to inject a very little amount of FAI compared to a higher dose of FAI required if I consume a high fast-acting carbohydrate (FAC) meal. And, if I am fasting, I take none FAI. So injecting a fixed pre-mixed dose of insulin is a complete non-sense and makes maneuverability and flexibility, between food and bolus insulin, almost impossible.

In addition, you can never use pre-mixed insulin to bring down a high blood sugar level. If you try this, your BS will go way down later on. You would not only inject short-acting insulin (the 30% part) but you would also inject intermediate-acting insulin (the 70% part). In brief, pre-mixed insulin gives you a rigid life filled with high and low numbers of blood sugar all the time. You sacrifice control and flexibility, which are two important keys to stable blood sugar and living well with diabetes.

Time to take the lead

My blood sugar numbers were constantly up and down with no solution offered by my physicians except *"this is diabetes and you have to accept it as it is"*. I refused that, enough is enough. After seven years of diagnosis, I was stifled and decided to search, read and find out myself how to control my BS. The search and luck led me to three great books. The first was Dr. Bernstein's book <u>Dr. Bernstein's Diabetes Solution</u>. The second was Gary Scheiner's book <u>Think Like a Pancreas</u>. And, finally, <u>Blood Sugar 101 What They Do Not Tell You About Diabetes,</u> by Jenny Ruhl rounded out my trio. These three great books led me to read about thirty more books in diabetes management, nutrition, obesity, brain health, cholesterol, fasting, and many other topics.

Initially, Dr. Bernstein, Gary Scheiner, and Jenny Ruhl books helped me to understand the science and math of MDI (multi-daily injections) along with understanding the effect of carbohydrate on blood sugar. I learned that it is possible to tightly control blood sugar with the approach of Dr. Bernstein by eating 30 grams of slow-acting carbohydrate (non-starchy vegetables) daily along with a sufficient amount of protein and a moderate amount of good fat. I also learned about insulin in terms of the right type, dosing, factors and timing. This was nothing short of magic to me considering the miserable fixed dose of pre-mixed insulin I was using at the time.

Besides reading and learning, I was also keen to practice and try everything day in and day out. I learned that I could never eat whatever I want and then inject for it if I had any hope of controlling my BS. If large amounts of fast-acting carbohydrates are eaten, many factors will jump in and make the BS control impossible.

However, before I reached this stage, I was completely influenced by Gary Scheiner's book Think Like a Pancreas and John Walsh, Varma, Roberts, Bailey book Using Insulin. I thought I could still eat any amount of FAC and match that with FAI injections if I only mastered insulin dosing and timing along with carbs' count.

Therefore, I started eating high whole carbs food and tried to maneuver around many factors such as:

- Calculating required bolus insulin units based on IC ratio.
- Where to inject.
- Type of insulin to be injected.
- The timing of injection-related to glycemic index and glycemic load of food eaten.
- Monitoring digestion pattern and assuming partial gastroparesis.
- Master carbohydrates count.

I tried numerous times to get a flat line of normal blood sugar but hell no; it was impossible. By doing so, there was no way to get my numbers where I wanted them at the normal range below 100 mg/dl or even below 120 mg/dl. Despite the unstable BS numbers resulted from my experiment but Somehow, I was satisfied that I proved to myself, the hard way though, this approach is not effective if I ever wanted real control of BS. I lost six more months of uncontrolled blood sugar but the lesson was worth it. You may ask, why did I want to achieve normal BS so badly? The simple answer is, I wanted to reverse some painful complications resulted from eight years of poor BS control and I knew that the only way to do it is to normalize my BS.

Now, after this practical experience, I heartily believed in the philosophy of Dr. Bernstein. I can sum it up as follows "it is impossible to match all mentioned factors together when adopting a high carbohydrate WOE."

I became fully dependent on insulin after eight years of diagnosis. I believe I needed insulin, starting the second year after diagnosis. I might preserve my remaining Beta cells if that happened. In fact, I am convinced that my type of diabetes is LADA, not T2 diabetic. In 2008, and after five years of uncontrolled BS, my first C peptide test put me in the lowest range of T1 diabetes. I am sure if the test was done second year after diagnosis, it would had shown a very less level of insulin as I was in continuous high BS regardless of any medicine or dose I took then. **This is a lesson for you; please ask for C peptide and insulin level tests to be done right after being diagnosed**.

After I admitted failure following in the mainstream approach, I started to see beautiful results of normal blood sugar following the low carb approach. In other words, Dr. Bernstein's approach. I was in total control of what I ate and what I got in my BS meter. It was like discovering an 8th Wonder of the World!

The one thing I regretted, I was not having this information before some complications had already started. However, I was fortunate enough to reverse most of them by keeping my BS in a normal range. For if you ask any mainstream physician, they will certainly tell you this is impossible.

The upshot is that controlling blood sugar is not an easy journey but it is possible. It needs efforts from your end; you need to be knowledgeable. You must learn and apply that on yourself. Choose the right physician who supports you and judges any approach only by results. Allow no one to dictate to you what to do when it comes to your blood sugar. Instead, be the master of your own version of diabetes. This is the only way, in my opinion, to achieve normal blood sugar and live peacefully with diabetes.

Chapter 2: Sad Reality

"To this day, the notion of treating diabetes by increasing consumption of the foods that caused the disease in the first place, then managing the blood sugar mess with medications, persists."
Dr. William Davis

I received a message on my FB diabetes page from Hosam (Not his real name), a 27 years old young man with T1 diabetes. He asked me desperately, "Why can't I control my blood sugar?" He had been T1 diabetic since he was 13; he has limited education and works a tough job that requires intense manual work for almost ten hours a day. His physician prescribed him pre-mixed insulin (30/70) and no matter what he does, he cannot control his BS with it. He can't follow low carb way of eating (WOE), as it is too expensive for him. Timidly, he admits that bread is the main part of his meals. He doesn't necessarily like it, but it is one of the few foods he can afford.

Hosam is a poor young man and he has no medical insurance. In his country, medical insurance is a luxury only for wealthy people! Sadly, he has already developed complications. He experiences such severe pins and needles sensation in his feet that sometimes stops him from going to work! Even thinking of MDI (Multiple-daily injections) option, using fast-acting and basal insulins is impossible, as he cannot afford to buy such expensive insulin.

My heart goes out to him. It seems unfair for a T1 young man to suffer like that while many people with diabetes in other countries get free insulin, insulin pump, and CGM by default and appears to take it for granted. CGM and pump are not even a dream for many PWD in poor parts of the world.

Hosam is not asking for fancy stuff. His humble wish is to be able to control his blood sugar with the proper insulin. He does not know about Xylitol, Erythritol, Swerve, Almond flour, Coconut flour, and Psyllium Husk. He doesn't know about Dexcom, Freestyle Libre, Enlite, Medtronic pumps, etc. He doesn't dare to dream about these luxuries. "My salary is equal to one kilogram of Almond flour," Hosam said in his message.

This is not an individual case; there are millions of people with diabetes out there in similar or even worse situations. Many of them can't even afford to buy the less expensive pre-mixed insulin. You find them in Africa, Asia, parts of the Middle East, parts of South America and many other countries.

These people do not have money to buy their medicine, insulin or even proper food to help them control their blood sugar. I know many friends in some countries who have no medical insurance. They have something similar to Medicaid in the USA. One person had to wait weeks for his insulin prescription to be approved. Imagine a person with T1 diabetes waiting that long without insulin. And, after all, they might decline his request for any trivial reason.

Similarly, many others forced by their countries' national medical insurance policies to use pre-mixed insulin only because it is cheaper. As I mentioned earlier, pre-mixed insulin makes it impossible for people with T1 diabetes to control BS. It reduces the ability to accurately match the insulin with the needs of the body. Because of this, the blood sugar often runs dangerously high. This quickly causes the devastating complications and severely reduces the quality of life of these unfortunate individuals.

Diabetes control should never be taken lightly. If I may, allow me to further illustrate the high cost of diabetes on human suffering. Almost half of all deaths attributable to high blood glucose occur before the age of 70. The World Health Organization (WHO) estimates that diabetes was the seventh leading cause of death in 2016. The number of people with diabetes has risen from 108 million in 1980 to 422 million in 2014. The global prevalence of diabetes among adults over 18 years of age has risen from 4.7% in 1980 to 8.5% in 2014! In 2016, an estimated 1.6 million deaths were caused by diabetes.[4]

Two third of the people with diabetes are of working age (327 Million). One million children have type one diabetes. Three-quarters of people with diabetes live in low or medium income countries (279 Million). These people live without proper management and suffer from the consequences of uncontrolled diabetes.

The total Number of Adults with diabetes is escalating from 151 Million in 2000 to 425 million in 2017 as shown in the picture from IDF 2017 Atlas.[5] As you can see, there is an unbelievable increase in the number of people diagnosed with diabetes year after year and yet there has been no real solution found out. This is especially true regarding dietary management.

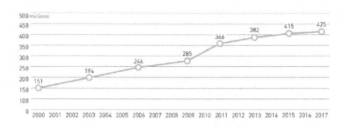

IDF Diabetes Atlas - 8th Edition

Let's take a closer look at a few specific examples from the IDF Diabetes Atlas fourth Edition to really understand the inequity of this sad reality.

Africa excluding Arab countries (IDF 2017 Atlas report):

Here the adult population is about **468** million and there are **15.5** million people diagnosed with diabetes between the ages of 20 to 79 years old. The percentage of undiagnosed people with diabetes is **69.2%** i.e. **10.7** million, and the annual death toll was estimated to be around **298,160** in 2017 (in which **77%** of them under the age of 60). The annual spending on diabetes treatment in this part of the world is **3.3** billion dollars. The number of children with T1 diabetes is **50,600.**[6]

North America and The Caribbean (NAC) (IDF 2017 Atlas report):

Here the adult population is **325** million and there are **45.9** million people diagnosed with diabetes between the ages of 20 to 79 years old. The percentage of undiagnosed people with diabetes is **37.6%** only i.e. **17.3** million and the annual death toll was estimated to be around **285,926** in 2017 (in which **36.9%** of them under the age of 60). The annual spending on diabetes treatment in this part of the world is **377.3** billion Dollars a year. The number of children with T1 diabetes is **216,300.**[7]

If we run a little comparison on the above two examples, we will simply notice the following:

1. Annual spending on diabetes treatment in NA and Caribbean (NAC) is almost **114 fold higher** than Africa.

2. The number of people diagnosed with diabetes in NAC is almost triple the number in Africa but the number of annual deaths is less in NA than in Africa!

3. The percentage of undiagnosed people with diabetes in Africa is almost double the percentage of NA.

4. The percentage of death below 60 years old in Africa is almost double the same percentage of NA.

5. Finally, despite the higher population in Africa as compared to NAC but the number of diagnosed T1 children in NAC is fourfold higher than Africa. In my opinion, this really needs to be investigated. What is the reason for this dramatic difference in the number of diagnosed T1 kids between NA and Africa? Is it the easy access to modern food, especially processed food? Is it Pollution, lack of sun exposure or immune system provocation? Is it the high number of undiagnosed T1 kids in Africa? Anyway, I doubt the latter could be the reason because T1 reveals itself so fast and it can't be left undiagnosed for a long time, unlike T2? Under any condition, I believe this phenomenon needs to be studied.

Even though the number of diagnosed people with diabetes (dd) in NAC is triple the number of dd in Africa, the annual death from diabetes in NAC is almost the same. Why? Notice the huge spending on diabetes treatment in NAC (114 fold). More specifically, note the lack of diabetes management spending in

Africa. This undeniably leads to severe complications, disability and the high percentage of death among people with diabetes in Africa.

When I see Africa statistics and when I receive a message like Hosam's one, some main questions pop up in my mind:

1. What are the moral obligations we, as people with diabetes, have towards the less fortunate people with diabetes all over the world?
2. How can we reach out to PWD such as Hosam and help them on the individual or organizational levels?
3. What are the contributions Big Pharma offering to help people who can't even afford insulin necessary for their survival?
4. How much from Big Pharma's profits has been contributed to support all the less fortunate PWD all over the world?
5. Why the price of a lifesaver medication like insulin is so ridiculously high?

I know there are many organizations out there trying to help, but this feels like a drop in the bucket compared to the huge numbers of people diagnosed every day and the huge number of people with horrible complications due to uncontrolled diabetes.

Let's get a better understanding of some of Big Pharma's profit. Examine carefully the global sales numbers of some famous diabetes drugs[8]:

1. Januvia sales in 2017 are 5.9 billion dollars.
2. Lantus sales in 2017 are 5.65 billion dollars.
3. Victoza sales in 2017 are 3.74 billion dollars.
4. Novorapid sales in 2017 are 3.23 billion dollars.
5. Humalog sales in 2017 are 2.87 billion dollars.
6. Levemir sales in 2017 are 2.28 billion dollars.

7. Trulicity sales in 2017 are 2.03 billion dollars.
8. Novomix 30 sales in 2017 are 1.65 billion dollars.
9. Humulin N sales in 2017 are 1.34 billion dollars.
10. Galvus sales in 2017 are 1.23 billion dollars.

If a very tiny fraction of these numbers were only spent to provide basic care to these unfortunate PWD in Africa and other similar countries, it would likely save tens of thousands of lives. We have not even yet considered the food industry. These businesses make billions of dollars of profit that are taken directly from the pockets of the poor who die daily, with hundreds, out of lack of medicine, medical care, and proper food.

If this situation is allowed to continue, these people are doomed to uncontrolled diabetes forever with painful and deadly complications. Proper insulin means life for people with T1 diabetes. It is not a luxury. Maybe the insulin pump and CGM (continuous glucose monitoring) are, but insulin is mandatory to all people with T1 diabetes and that has to be afforded without a question. Until this happens, the HbA1c of 5% or even 7% stays a dream impossible to be achieved to Hosam and the like all over the world. That is such a sad reality indeed.

Chapter 3: My Meter is My Approval

"The resistance of the medical profession to dietary carbohydrate restriction in the treatment of metabolic syndrome and, more important, to its most obvious risk, diabetes, I find incomprehensible."

Richard David Feinman

The legendary Diabetologist Dr. Richard Bernstein said, "My insistence is that People with diabetes are entitled to the same normal blood sugar that Non-Diabetics enjoy rather than ADA's current insistence upon higher levels."[9] This quote sums it all up. It changed my approach in dealing with diabetes. I do not settle for less with diabetes anymore because I know that diabetes will never settle for less with me. And, I know that I deserve to live my life with normal blood sugar even if I am a diabetic. One of my dreams is that I could live to witness the day that all endocrinologists think the same way towards PWD.

My HbA1c remained in the range between 8 and 11 for eight years because I carefully followed the advice of my physician. This advice was not unique to my physician. This was, and still is, the standard advice received from nearly all mainstream physicians.

When I first read <u>Dr. Bernstein's Diabetes Solution,</u> I thought, "How different this book is from conventional mainstream advice." However, when I followed his suggestions, I got instant improvement in my blood sugar numbers. In fact, my numbers were not just improved, they were near NORMAL. After years of struggling on the mainstream advice, this seemed to happen virtually overnight. By the way, there is no magic in what Dr. Bernstein preaches about. It is just a common sense equation; stop eating the food that raises your blood sugar in the first place, then you will be able to control your BS. That is it.

By following his wisdom, your results can also be far from mediocre. Your blood sugar will improve dramatically by just cutting out starches, grains, sugars, juices, sodas, and fruits except for berries. Your need for insulin will be decreased by a large percentage if you are T1 and you might never have to use it if you are T2. It is amazing how these sustainable small changes could lead to great results if we are committed.

The nagging questions are:

Why does nobody care as much as Dr. Bernstein?

If such an approach could lead to such magnificent results, so why do endocrinologists not follow the same path? Or else figure out another path to lead to normal blood sugar if they do not like his way!

Can't the mainstream physicians notice what is going on with their diabetes patients and how soon, after diagnosis, they suffer from these terrifying complications?

Can't they see their patients follow their guidelines and still achieve HbA1c's of 8, 9, 10 and above?

Can't they see the consistent high blood sugar numbers and its constant fluctuations?

Can't they see many of their patients are on dialysis, have poor vision or suffer from sleep deprivation due to neuropathic pain? Why do they ignore this misery?

Are the amputations, blindness, kidney failure, and cardiovascular damage not enough for them to adopt a paradigm shift? What else is needed for them to save PWD from such slow and agonizing path to death?

Why don't they change their approach towards diabetes management? Why they do not challenge the conventional wisdom of ADA, and likes?

And, why don't they spend more efforts to support the patients in achieving real control of diabetes: the level of control that protects them from the deadly complications?

Nine months ago, a friend of mine noticed an acute onset of continuous thirst and frequent urination. He visited his physician, who ordered some lab's works. Two of the requested lab's work were: glucose intolerance test (GIT) and fasting blood sugar test (FBT). The results were as follows: GIT 198 mg/dl after one hour, 166 mg/dl after two hours and FBT was 123 mg/dl. To my amazement, his Dr. advised him to stick to a low fat diet, high in whole grains! Unbelievable!

The advice given to my friend; was also given to me for 8 years and continues to be given to countless others every day around the globe. That fills me with sadness and anger because I believe many of those poor souls will return back to their careless physicians in a year or two with full-blown diabetes with numbers like 400 mg/dl or higher, as it was for me.

For a moment, let's assume this physician told my friend, "Unfortunately you are diabetic but the good news is, you could easily reverse it. You need to act immediately by cutting sugars, starches and starting to exercise." What do you think the outcome will be? I think the whole future of my friend would be brighter.

Luckily, my friend told me the story and I referred him to Dr. Bernstein book so he can get the right advice. Guess what? Just by opting to the proper dietary choice, he lost 35 pounds and his HbA1c now is 5.1. His blood sugar never exceeds 110 mg/dl around the clock. What a difference!

It is so sad to see PWD, needlessly, suffer especially when there are successful alternatives explained in details by many respected and proactive physicians, scientists, nutritionists or diabetes educators. I will mention some of the names that make a positive difference in a world full of valueless guidelines: Dr. Bernstein, Dr. David Perlmutter, Gary Taubes, Dr. William Davis, Maria Emmerich, Dr. Peter Attia, Dr. Richard Feinman, Dr. David Ludwig, Dr. Jason Fung, Dr. Eric Westman, Dr. Gary Fettke, Franziska Spritzler, Dr. Tom Noakes and others.

The majority of physicians appear to turn a blind eye on this ongoing suffering. Why? Is it because of ego, misplaced fear, or business considerations? In fact, big organizations' guidelines inhibit physicians from adopting such approaches under the guise of moderation; justified by one pacifying infamous phrase "everyone is different".

Look at what happened in South Africa to prof. Tim Noakes, who is one of the world brilliancies in his specialty. He was charged with misconduct by the Health Professional Council of South Africa (HPCSA), just because he advised a mother to wean her child onto a low carb high fat food, in twitter! In the end, he won the three years brutal battle but the message of terrorizing and silencing of whoever dares to say the truth had reached many physicians all around the world.

"I was put on the stand for nine days. I didn't have to retract a single thing. I'm probably the first scientist who has had to defend their beliefs under oath since Galileo," Dr. Noakes said.

Australian orthopedic surgeon Dr. Gary Fettke is another great doctor who refused to be bullied. The Australian Health Practitioners Regulatory Authority (AHPRA) silenced him. He was told not to give any nutritional advice to his diabetic patients! As Marika Sboros said it perfectly *"Australian orthopedic surgeon Dr. Gary Fettke can no longer advise his diabetic patients on nutrition to prevent limb amputation. In particular, he cannot tell patients not to eat sugar."*

AHPRA stated, *"There is nothing associated with your medical training or education that makes you an expert or authority in the field of nutrition, diabetes or cancer. Even if, in the future, your views on the benefits of the LCHF lifestyle become the accepted best medical practice this does not change the fundamental fact that you are not suitably trained or educated as a medical practitioner to be providing advice or recommendations on this topic."*

In other words, Dr. Feinman says, *"Credentials are more important than the truth."*[10]

After 4.5 years of bitter battle, AHPRA dropped all charges against Dr. Gary. They cleared him from misconduct and wrongdoing. In fact, he received an official apology letter from AHPRA. Dr. Gary was, unbelievably, supported by his great wife Belinda Fettke. Indeed, It is an honor to me that Dr. Gary wrote me the foreword of this book. You can read more about his story on www.isupportgary.com

The stories of Dr. Noakes and Dr. Fettke show us to what extent brave physicians could be bullied and terrorized by big medical organizations. This kind of actions let many physicians think more than twice before saying the truth. Therefore, the sentence "everyone is different" became an easy excuse for many physicians to justify sticking to the guidelines, so they will not be hurt and victimized.

In your journey with diabetes, you need to find a brave doctor just like Dr. Noakes and Gary. Doctors who say the truth no matter how bad the consequences. Those are the real heroes indeed. Unfortunately, they are hard to find but not impossible, if you search patiently.

When it comes to diabetes management, I partially agree that everyone is different and requires a unique regimen. However, I also feel strongly that everyone is entitled to normal blood sugar and the level of carbohydrates intake should be adjusted to achieve that end.

For me, I decided long ago, I needed neither an organization nor a physician to tell me which blood sugar numbers are good to follow. I realized that my prime concern is to achieve normal blood sugar at any cost, regardless of who advises the contrary. Moreover, I made anything leads to normalizing my BS, a priority in my life.

I opt for healthy food choices, small food portions, weight reduction, exercising, fasting, and frequent blood sugar monitoring. Then I use whatever medicine needs to be used to keep normal blood sugar (described by a knowledgeable doctor). I only stick to what brings good results.

My meter becomes my approval. My meter is my evidence, and my BS numbers will always be my Judge. I was once sinking to the bottom of this Rough Ocean called diabetes and Dr. Bernstein's advice saved me and brought me up to the surface where I can now swim and breathe. Following his simple and common sense approach took me from HbA1c of 10 to HbA1c of 5.5.

Thanks to Dr. Richard Bernstein, the brilliant engineer who became a great physician! What he taught me has saved my life and lives of thousands of other People with diabetes. And, thanks for every proactive doctor who thinks outside of the box and makes a difference in the lives of others.

Chapter 4: The Low Carb approach and a Coffee without Sugar!

"Spill Butter on the floor – slip. Spill fruit juice on the floor – sticky. Same goes for your arteries."
Gary Fettke.

D iabetes can simply be defined as the inability of the body to deal with carbohydrates. As carbohydrates are digested into glucose, it is essentially the inability of the body to deal efficiently with glucose. Most body cells require insulin to utilize glucose as energy. In both pre-diabetes and T2 diabetes, cells become resistant to insulin. This is seen as a measure of protection against the toxic effect of high blood glucose.

In T1 diabetes, the immune system attacks pancreatic beta cells (insulin-producing cells). Therefore, there is little or no insulin production to deal with blood glucose resulting from food digestion. In both cases, the end result is high blood sugar.

Hence, in all cases mentioned above, the first line of any approach to successful diabetes management has to start with reducing the entry of glucose to the body as much as possible. Physicians prohibit salt from the person with high blood pressure, gluten from the person with Celiac disease, and peanuts from someone with peanut allergy. So why the same is not considered with carbohydrates intake for people with diabetes?

To manage diabetes successfully, carbohydrates restriction is not only common sense; it is the optimal approach and should be tried first. Dr. Richard David Feinman calls it *"The default approach,"* in his book The World Turned Upside Down. The Low carbohydrates approach (LC) is one of the main strategies leads to achieve normal blood sugar along with the appropriate oral medication or proper insulin therapy if required.

Unfortunately, this fact is been overlooked by most of the people dealing with diabetes from the medical field whether they are physicians, nutritionists or diabetes educators. They may advise you to stop eating sugar and, of course, fat. When they say sugar, they actually mean the white table sugar and sweets. Some of them may be a little more restrictive and ask you to refrain from not only white sugar but also from processed wheat. However, very few will talk to you about the huge effect of whole grains on your blood sugar and fructose on your triglyceride numbers. In fact, whole grains are considered "healthy" by the diet-heart hypothesis (low fat paradigm). The mainstream medicine continues to be resistant to low carb diets despite the mounting evidence in the medical literature about this way of eating (WOE).

It is not a coincidence that the rate of obesity and the prevalence of diabetes have risen in epidemic proportions when the consumption of these foods has increased since the mid-eighties when the low fat paradigm was king.

I contend that low fat, high carbohydrate paradigm is not only responsible for the epidemic spread of diabetes, but it is also the main culprit of uncontrolled diabetes among PWD. By logic, if high carb diet raises blood sugar, so it will also be responsible for the inevitable health deterioration and progression of severe complications accompany the diagnosis.

Why do physicians reject this WOE!?

The American Diabetes Association (ADA) is the organization that puts forth the treatment guidelines for the people with diabetes in the US. This is followed not only by physicians in the US but likely by physicians in most parts of the world. Sadly, people think that if they follow these guidelines, they will control their blood sugar and avoid complications. In my opinion, two main recommendations of the ADA have devastating consequences to the health of people with diabetes.

First: The ADA sets blood sugar target far from normal. Physicians teach these goals to PWD all over the world. Take a look at the BS target mentioned in ADA 2016 guidelines:

- Postprandial (after food), under 180 mg/dL.
- Pre-prandial (before food), between 80 to 130 mg/dL.
- HbA1c under 7%.[11]

In fact, sticking to such high BS goal has caused the diabetes complications rate to rise globally among PWD. Remember, these goals are being pushed and adopted by almost all physicians. I was one of those ADA blood sugar's target followers before I adopted normal blood sugar as my goal.

Second: ADA recommends that the person with diabetes eat about 45 to 60 grams of carbohydrates per meal. They believe complex carbohydrates such as whole wheat bread, brown rice, whole-wheat pasta, bulgur, and oats are healthy carbohydrates for people with diabetes to consume freely. Unfortunately, this cannot be further from the truth. To be honest, ADA recently changed its stance, partially, about the low carb WOE and said that it could be beneficial to people with T2 diabetes but ADA still says that low carb approach is hard to be followed! More details about the new ADA statement in chapter 15.

The myth of whole wheat

Unfortunately, one of the most prevailing myths in diabetes management and obesity is the "so-called" healthy whole grain bread or brown bread. Many nutritionists claim that it has a slower impact in raising blood sugar that it is well tolerated by people with diabetes. This is not right at all.

Let me explain to you why the brown bread raises blood sugar of PWD faster than bananas, chocolate, and white sugar. In the words of Dr. David Perlmutter, the author of the beautiful book <u>Grain Brain</u>: *"in many medical conferences, I used to ask the following question for each of those present and usually all are working in the medical field: Which one of the following food raises blood sugar fastest? Brown bread (healthy as we think), bananas, chocolate or white sugar?"* said Dr. Perlmutter.

"In 99% of cases the answer comes wrong; either bananas or chocolate or sugar, but no one ever says brown bread! "The truth is that brown bread is the owner of the highest glycemic index among any of these foods mentioned above!" said Dr. Perlmutter.[12] For your information, the glycemic index is a ranking of food according to their effect on your blood sugar. The higher the rank, the faster and higher this food will raise your blood sugar.

Both brown bread and white bread are processed and stripped from all possible nutrients, which left them with starch, gluten, and some fiber. Dr. Perlmutter used an entire book to demonstrate the harms gluten does to our bodies and to our brains in specific. The only difference between white and brown bread is that the latter has some extra fiber in it which delaying the sugar absorption in intestines by about ten to twenty minutes. However, the grams of carbohydrate content is almost equal for the same weight of bread whether it is white or whole wheat.

Therefore, if I, as an insulin-dependent diabetic, eat brown bread instead of white bread of the same weight, I will inject the same units of fast-acting insulin but with a slight adjustment in timing. In other words, if I inject insulin 20 minutes before eating the white bread, I will inject it 10 minutes before eating whole wheat bread. This is the only difference.

A large Pita bread 6 ½ inches in diameter, 60 grams in weight contains 33 grams of fast-acting carbohydrates (FAC) in it. In many parts of the world PWD eat at least 2 pitas each meal, (i.e. 66 grams of FAC/meal). That is equal to about 16.5 teaspoons of sugar in grams of carbohydrate count, as each teaspoon of sugar has 4 grams of carbs in it! The sole difference between pita and sugar is that all the carbs' grams in the bread will turn to glucose in your body, while table sugar has 50% glucose and 50% Fructose. The glucose goes directly to the bloodstream through intestines. While the fructose does not raise blood sugar but on the other side, it turns to triglyceride in the liver which causes many damages, one of which is fatty liver.

One gram of FAC raises the blood sugar of 150 lb non-obese T1 diabetic adult man about 5 mg/dl. This 66 gm of carbohydrates in these two pitas are supposed to raise this person's blood sugar about 330 mg/d. Assuredly, the blood sugar rise will peak in about 45 minutes. Thus, **if you are a person with T1 Diabetes**, you need to inject early enough before eating the bread and you will require an enormous amount of insulin to cover this flood of ingested glucose. From my own experience, I never controlled my BS while eating bread.

If you are T2, you will secret a huge amount of valuable insulin that may not adequately cover the rise in blood sugar. In part, this is due to insulin resistance, the delayed release of insulin and insufficient phase 1 insulin production in T2 diabetics. This amount of insulin either injected or secreted in T1 or T2 respectively, will cause instability and extensive fluctuations of blood sugar. Additionally, in T2 case, this will definitely lead to further exhaustion of the already exhausted beta cells.

A common sense equation:
Fast-acting Carbohydrates = more insulin secreted and medication is taken for T2 (or more insulin injected for T1) = resistance to insulin = overweight = continuous hunger = More

food and insulin needed = Uncontrolled blood sugar. IT IS A VICIOUS CIRCLE.

To make it more comprehensible, let me put it that way: As an insulin user, I will inject one unit of fast insulin if I consume one spoon of sugar but I will inject eight units of insulin if I eat these two pieces of pita bread. This is for the sake of comparison and not to say, "Eat sugar."

Elaborating more, I want you to imagine if you as a person with diabetes eat six of the Pita bread daily (two every meal). That is nearly 200 grams of carbohydrates. This means you almost ate 50 teaspoons of sugar that day (remember a teaspoon of sugar has 4 grams of carbs). I did not even consider any other sugary or starchy food you may have eaten throughout the day such as rice, potatoes, fruits, pasta or sweet. Any of these would easily raise up your daily intake of sugar to about 100 spoons a day.

Bread (wheat) is converted to glucose in your body massively and rapidly. This is a well-known scientific fact for decades. Somehow, this idea has been let go. I suspect it is for the sake of pharma and food businesses. Many respectable physicians and scientists have written about this fact in many books. Let me note some of these books here in case if you are interested to learn more:

- Grain Brain by Dr. David Perlmutter.
- Wheat Belly by Dr. William Davis.
- Dr. Richard Bernstein's Diabetes Solution by Dr. Richard Bernstein.
- Blood sugar 101 by Jenny Ruhl.
- The Truth about Low Carb diet by Jenny Ruhl.
- Why We Get Fat and what we can do about it by Gary Taubes.
- Good Calories Bad Calories by Gary Taubes.
- Keto-Adapted by Maria Emmerich.
- Low Starch Diabetes Solution by Dr. Rob Thompson.
- The World Turned Upside Down by Dr. Richard David Feinman.

- Why We Are Hungry by Dr. David Ludwig.
- The Low Carb Dietitian's Guide to Health and Beauty by Franziska Spritzler.
- The Obesity Code by Dr. Jason Fung.
- Diabetes Code by Dr. Jason Fung.
- The Complete Guide To Fasting by Dr. Jason Fung.

Ironically, most physicians advise PWD to drink tea or coffee without sugar. While they do not even tell them about the crazy effect of bread, rice, juice or pasta on their blood sugar.

Many PWD have no clue about the harmful effect of fast-acting carbohydrates on their BS. So, they think by cutting sugar only, everything should be fine. They eat starches on a daily basis and ask the following questions, without knowing that the sole answer is to quit this kind of food:

- Why are we so hungry all the time?
- Why are our brains foggy?
- Why is our energy always depleted?
- Where has this belly come from?
- Why have we gotten T2 diabetes?
- Why are our kids getting so fat?
- Why are so many kids being diagnosed with T2 diabetes at very early ages?
- And, the big question is: why is my HbA1c 9 or 10, although we drink coffee without sugar?!

In summary, when I cut all fast-acting carbohydrates, I was able to reduce my bolus insulin about 70% and my basal about 20%. NOW MULTIPLY ME BY MILLIONS OF PWD all over the world. If everyone followed the same approach and cut the sugar and starches, it will be disastrous for Big Pharma and Grains Industry. Perhaps now you can understand why they fight this WOE so aggressively. It will definitely create a huge drop in insulin, drugs and wheat/corn sales and profits. And to be honest, This is why I think the guidelines, we talked about, will not be changed soon.

Chapter 5: Hamza and the Mixtard

"In some sense, the problem with convincing people of the benefits of a reduced carbohydrate strategy is that it appears to be good for everything, good for what ails you. You can sound like a hard-sell pitchman."
Richard David Feinman

I was ruminating on the business trip I was about to start. It was a long five hours overnight flight. I spent the time between taking a short nap, reading and listening to some music. I reached my destination and grabbed my bags. As soon as my feet touched the land of the beautiful city of Koshi, India, I was fascinated by the pouring rain.

It was raining, as I have never seen before in my whole life. That rain was powerful yet charming. A kind of rain that cleans you from the inside out. I just let my soul sailing along with the flow of God's beauty and enjoyed the pure smell of the rainwater when it mixes with the grassy ground! The idea that the rain is free for every creature to use always inspires me. Rain voluntarily serves all of us. **It has always taught me to serve without expecting something in return.**

Standing outside the arrival terminal under the shed, amazed by the marvelous scene of the heavy rain, I felt a hand touching my shoulder gently and a voice asking, "Are you Eng. Ahmed?" I said "yes."

He said, "I am Hamza".

Mr. Hamza is a sixty years old Indian man with a medium white beard. His face reveals his kindness and tells how an easy-going character he is. I also noticed some kind of pallor and paleness in his face, that kind of paleness I know well!

Hamza took me to the hotel promising he would come back tomorrow to discuss our business issues. I tried to get a little nap but I couldn't. I was kind of tottering between being so tired and not able to sleep. From the comfort of the hotel room, I sent my eyes to follow the giant raindrops as they slid rapidly down the window panes. I made a cup of black tea and I sat behind the window, humbled I was allowed to enjoy such a beautiful scene. Ultimately, I slept like a baby on the rhythm of the raindrops music. Next morning, I met Hamza, and he drove me directly to his office.

Hamza watched me measuring my blood sugar three times in about 7 hours. The first time he saw me measuring my blood sugar, he just ignored it. Then the second time he was looking at me the "are you crazy" look. And, the third time he came out of his silence and said loudly, "Mr. Ahmed, are you crazy? You have measured your blood sugar three times in six or seven hours?"

I smiled and answered, "Mr. Hamza, the moment I saw you, I knew you are diabetic. And I also knew you don't control your blood sugar; Am I right?" I asked.

"Yes I am diabetic but you were wrong about uncontrolled diabetes. I am controlling my BS very well my friend," Hamza said.

"Fine Hamza, how many times you measure your BS daily," I replied immediately.

Hamza, indignantly, "Daily! I measure my BS once a month as per my doctor Instructions and I do this in his clinic in my monthly visit there!"

"Ok, and what is your usual reading in this once-a-month measurement Mr. Hamza?" I replied.

"Between 190 to 250 mg/dl, two hours after food," Hamza replied with confidence.

"And what did your Dr. tell you about these BS numbers Hamza?" I asked.

"Nothing. He just advised me to walk 30 minutes a day," Hamza replied.

"What medication are you taking Mr. Hamza?" I asked.

"Pre-mixed Insulin 30 – 70," Hamza said.

OMG, again the pre-mixed insulin! We have discussed how many physicians in this part of the world and actually in the US as well, keep prescribing it to make it easy for themselves. By doing so, they can avoid explaining things like correction factors, carb factor, carb calculation, basal adjustment, etc. They simply recommend fixed morning and night doses. In my opinion, it is impossible to control blood sugar with pre-mixed insulin. One of the big lessons I learned and helped me control my BS was to think like a Pancreas, which is spelled out as in Gary Scheiner's book Think Like a Pancreas.

"Mr. Hamza, can you please measure your BS now?" I asked.

"Of course, give me a minute," Hamza replied with confidence.

It was 292 mg/dl! Hamza was shocked, but I wasn't. I know how the control with pre-mixed insulin is, as I had been there for two years before I learned how to own back my destiny. I also watched Hamza having a breakfast of two big pieces of bread with lentils.

"Do you have any of the diabetes complications Mr. Hamza?" I asked.

"Yes Ahmed I do, my feet hurt with pinning all the time and sex with my wife had become a thing from the past. That all started about three years ago," Hamza replied timidly, trying to avoid eye contact.

"And what did your Dr. tell you about this Hamza?" I asked.

"Nothing, he just said, this is the nature of diabetes, it is a progressive disease," Hamza replied.

"Hamza, answer me honestly, do you really want to control your blood sugar?" I asked.

"Of course," Hamza confirmed.

"Then listen carefully my friend," I replied. Then I elaborated immediately and started to explain about insulin and food skills. We talked about IC ratio, correction factors, IOB calculation, carbohydrate counting, and fast-acting insulin function. I explained the importance of basal insulin, how to master MDI, how to decide the numbers of FAI units required for food. We spoke about the correction method of high and low BS and the difference between fast-acting and slow-acting carbohydrate. And, I evoked the story of Dr. Bernstein and his approach. In the end, I looked at Hamza straight in the eye and said, "here is a big surprise my friend; the most important thing that will enable you to control your BS."

Hamza opened his mouth surprisingly and said, "What will be that?"

"With such breakfast, there will be no BS control. As of now NO WHEAT, NO GRAINS, NO SUGAR, less fruits, and no Juices. THEY ARE ALL PURE GLUCOSE IN YOUR BLOOD. Keeping a normal blood sugar is the only way could help you to have sex again with your wife Mr. Hamza." I said.

"What! Pure sugar! How come my Dr. never warned from such food especially wheat!" Hamza replied with a denying voice.

"Hold on a second Ahmed, if you allow me, as I am so confused. This is a big subject and I need more time to comprehend. First, let me take you back to the hotel and I will bring my son (I knew he is an engineer later) and come over to you this evening to chat about all this in details again. PLEASE HELP ME," Hamza said.

"OK Mr. Hamza, Take me to the hotel and I will be ready for you this evening," I replied while talking to myself "diabetes follows me wherever I go, amazing!"

I arrived at the hotel at 6 pm, took a shower, got ready and Hamza came at 7 pm as promised. We met at the lobby, drank coffee together and I started taking all his questions one by one and answering them clearly with a background sound of pouring rain again. I made it clear for him that first, he must look for a knowledgeable physician and consult with him about all we had discussed. I also advised him to read Dr. Bernstein's book.

He kept asking about everything repeatedly and I answered them all. Meanwhile, I was writing everything down for him, as he requested. While I was writing, I raised my head and looked at him and to my amazement; his tears were flowing down his eyes while his face turned red.

"What happened Hamza?" I asked.

He said, "You know what Ahmed, My office is in Koshi but I live 200 Km away from here. In fact, I was not supposed to attend this business trip with you. My elder son was the one supposed to meet you, but he got terrible flu two days ago and I replaced him to be with you. My sweet fate led me here to meet with you, perhaps, to save my life. This is God's work. Not me not you." Hamza said with misty eyes while looking up to the sky.

"I have five diabetic people in my close family, their conditions just like me, and I will learn, practice and help them if I can," Hamza said.

We sat together until 2 am and I gave him a complete guide of real diabetes management for his coming years. I summed it all up for him. Before he left, I emphasized, again, about the importance of finding a supporting and knowledgeable doctor.

I got back to my room exhausted, but also so complacent and calm. Sleep was gone but I was happy and that is what matters. **Real happiness comes along with supporting people without waiting for anything in return, Just like RAIN.**

Next morning at 6 am, Hamza picked me up to the airport, walked me towards departure hall, and hugged me an emotional long goodbye hug. We both were tearing just like the nonstop rain outside. What a beautiful state of mind my memory will carry for a long time.

On the way to the airport, Hamza told me he bought the required basal and fast-acting Insulin and started the no grain no wheat way of eating this very morning's breakfast itself. He looked at me straight in the eye and said, "There will be no way back what so ever."

Some hours later, I arrived at the Dubai airport to find an SMS that deeply touched my heart and brought tears again to my red eyes. SMS said, "Dear Ahmed, you are God's gift sent to me. For the first time in 11 years, being T2 and insulin-dependent diabetic, I measured 118 mg/dl two hours after food, I can't believe it. I just want to thank you a million and thank GOD I met you." A trip I will never forget.

Chapter 6: I cannot stop eating – The Leptin resistance

"It is difficult to get a man to understand something, when his salary depends on his not understanding it. – Upton Sinclair, American writer" — Tim Noakes, Lore of Nutrition

I want you to ponder a little about the beautiful experience of living without this crazy urge for food all the time. My aim of this book is not to tell you what to eat or how much you are supposed to eat, as I am not a nutritionist. My aim is to draw your attention to be more alert towards what you eat because the right selection of food is your first line of defence while managing diabetes. My intention is to inform you how eliminating some foods made the huge difference in controlling my appetite and my blood sugar once and forever. I believe this will do the same for you as well. However, I feel this cannot be dictated as it is something you must go through yourself. Once you have experienced the positive difference, it becomes impossible to ignore.

Opting for the right healthy food is a crucial element in achieving normal blood sugar. Unfortunately, it seems many people with diabetes lack this skill. One of the main things helped me normalize my blood sugar was that I learned how to be cautious with food choices and how to control my desire to eat all the time, which is common in people with diabetes and prediabetes. So, how did this habit of increased food consumption developed? To answer this question, please allow me to elaborate on the glorification of the culture of eating without limits in our societies.

In our human history, we have never experienced such a time where the food is abundant and obtainable in such the way as it is now. In fact, we have become eating machines. We do not eat to live anymore, but we live to eat. Our culture has become full of occasions that we directly connect to food consumption. You name it: Thanksgiving, Christmas, Halloween, Passover, Ramadan feast (Eid), Ramadan itself, Adha Eid in Muslims tradition, etc.

Most family gatherings are centered on food consumption in one way or another. Our predilection with food becomes phenomenal. We love to eat; we establish all possible rituals that lead us to consume plenty of food all the time without even thinking about whether we are really hungry.

We create an ongoing environment that invites us to gulp food. Giants food and beverages corporations surround us by intoxicating artificial food aromas, cooking TV programs, delicious recipes, endless fast-food chains, the culture of indulging in baked food/sweets/donuts, giant street images of food dishes, fatty food, starchy food, juice, Coca Cola, Pepsi, beer, large/double burgers, combo orders, big sizes of fast food, "extra size it" French fries and more. Food manufacturers add artificial colors, aromas, flavors, and taste to our kids' food so they can be addicted to the taste, smell and shape. They fake the flavor via all these foods science and marketing tricks to get customers to try all the fake foods on hypermarkets shelves. When all these influences are mixed together, we end up eating high carbs, high protein, high sugar, high fructose, high fructose corn syrup, and high fat food altogether in one table.

Moreover, we sentimentalize food in our movies by squeezing many scenes within the scenario of:

- Family gathering around a nice dining table full of food.
- A couple going out to have dinner or lunch in a fancy restaurant.
- Business meetings around the food table.

And, while watching movies, joy can't be completed without a huge popcorn and giant Cola! You see scenes of food in your real-life, social media and on TV maybe over 10 times a day, which turns on your desire to try all these food varieties. In addition, thanks to modern transportation, that enables us to find any kind of food at any time of the year regardless of its planting and harvest times. If you live in a hot country where the temperature reaches 105 f in summer, you still can eat salmon comes to you directly from Alaska. The opposite is true, if you live in Alaska, you can get mango, papaya, and pineapple coming to your table from Sri Lanka or the Philippines 365 days a year.

In addition, we also get the wrong nutritional advice. Our nutritionists keep us in a continuous feeding state by recommending eating three meals a day along with a couple of snacks. We have even invented another name for a meal between breakfast and lunch "brunch!"

Continuous feeding vs controlled feeding is another example, parallel to the diabetes example, where going the opposite direction of mainstream advice, makes a big difference. Rather than feeding into this constant appetite as suggested by nutritionists, I am talking about the use of fasting. Intermittent fasting is a major approach used by many throughout the ages. Dr. Jason Fong uses this approach in reversing T2 diabetes. In other words, the reduction of food consumption along with better choices of food will play a vital role in your diabetes management. While Dr. Fung, mainly talks about type 2 diabetes, intermittent fasting shows fruitful results with insulin-dependent type 1 diabetes as well.

Remarkably, many people with diabetes and even non-diabetics (especially overweight ones) have an increased appetite for food. Their brain no longer receives the satiety signal to stop the continuous desire for eating. Most likely, this happens because of "Leptin resistance".

In one study included newly diagnosed sixty T2 patients, found that hyperleptinemia, reflecting leptin resistance and lead to insulin resistance.[13] In fact, both lead to each other.

Leptin Story

Leptin is a hormone produced by fat cells to signal the brain they are full. Upon receiving the signal, the brain transmits back signals to the body to stop eating and start raising the metabolic rate. Therefore, when you are leptin sensitive, you could burn your fat easier, feel full faster and enjoy high metabolic rate. But, when you are leptin resistant, your brain does not get the required Leptin signal. As a result, the brain refrains from giving the three big commands:

1. Stop eating.
2. Stop storing energy as fat.
3. Increase the metabolic rate.

Instead, it induces the body to eat more, store more fat and to slow the metabolic rate, as he thinks you are starving.

Insulin resistance

Scientists say, leptin resistance goes hand in hand with Insulin resistance, which is caused by many factors. An overweight T2 diabetic or non-diabetic, most likely suffer from both insulin and Leptin resistance. This assumption is mostly correct if they couldn't lose weight easily, no matter what approach they took.

There are many reasons behind insulin resistance but the major contributor to insulin resistance is the high level of insulin secreted due to eating a lot of starchy, sugary food, fructose, and high fructose corn Syrup. As we know, higher blood glucose is poisonous to our bodies. Therefore, body cells resist insulin to stop the extra glucose from entering them. Accordingly, the pancreas secretes more insulin to push the extra glucose into cells to clear bloodstream from it. *The more you produce insulin, the more your body will resist it.*

On the other hand, fructose goes directly from intestines to the liver and gets converted to triglyceride. Production of triglycerides and subsequent storage of fat in the liver leads to fatty liver and the storage of visceral fat (internal fat storage around organs), both which contributes further to insulin resistance. Therefore, white table sugar has a double negative effect on your insulin sensitivity. Sugar contains 50% glucose and 50% fructose and, HFCS (high fructose corn syrup) is 55% fructose and 45% glucose. The glucose in these common forms of sugar raises the blood sugar and accordingly raises insulin level while the fructose is converted to triglyceride. Both high insulin level and TG lead to insulin resistance. So, if you follow a high carb WOE, you open up several roads that lead to insulin resistance. **It is only when I stopped eating starches and fructose, my crazy TG numbers (600 to 1200 range) went down to below 120 mg/dl and my insulin resistance was dramatically improved.**

When you eat a lot of sugary and starchy food in a repeated daily pattern, your insulin fluctuates. By the time insulin level goes down, another hormone called Ghrelin (the hunger hormone) goes up causing you to be hungry and eat again. Then you are into an endless vicious circle. The circle that will put fat around your waist, but especially around your internal organs as visceral fat. Both body fat and visceral fat make your cells insulin resistant and again cause Leptin resistance!

In brief, the more we consume food that turns to glucose inside our bodies; the more we secrete insulin and the more we become insulin resistant. This applies to Leptin and Leptin resistance as well. In addition, the more fructose we eat, the more fat we store and the more insulin and leptin resistant we become.

What about hunger?

In his book <u>The Complete guide to fasting</u> Dr. Jason Fung said that hunger is a mental state; not a stomach state. He said, *"Hunger, obviously, is not simply a reflection of the amount of food filling our stomach. Instead, hunger is partly a learned phenomenon. Even when we don't think we are hungry, smelling a steak and hearing it sizzle may make us quiet ravenous."*[14] That is true, sometimes I pass by a restaurant and smell the Shish Kabab I like and instantly I crave the Kabab although I am full. The mental hunger is working here not the physical one.

That is why fasting is a good exercise to differentiate between real hunger and an imaginary one. Let me give you a real-life example here again. In Ramadan, Muslims fast from dawn to sunset, which is around 16 hours. Neither food nor drinks are allowed before sunset. Ramadan meant to let people feel the poor who cannot afford to eat even once a day. Unfortunately, many people eat excessively during the nights of Ramadan after breaking their fast. It was never meant to be the month of food gulping from sunset until dawn!

Based on my personal experience of Ramadan fasting, I could differentiate between mental and physical hunger, passing the fifth or sixth day of fasting. This is especially true if I break my fast away from sugary and starchy food. Fasting suppresses my hunger as my body adapts to nutritional ketosis (burning the fat as fuel instead of glucose). Passed day 6, I lose the 3 pm screaming hunger signal in my stomach.

Unfortunately, Ramadan, for many, has become the month of getting heavier, higher blood sugar, higher Triglyceride and amazingly it has become the month of higher food bills although we abstain from food almost ¾ the day.

What to do?

So, how can we come out of this culture of extensive food consumption whether or not we have diabetes? I will share with you what to do based on my experience. Of course, this is not the only way to do it. I just share my successful experience and the choice is yours. I recommend you to go through the next two steps :

The first step you need to focus more on food choices. Target adequate protein from natural sources (Grass-fed cows for example) with whatever natural fat comes with it, along with leafy vegetables. Dr. Bernstein said, *"For a sedentary person we use 1.2 g protein per every Kg of body weight (.55 g/lb) as a starting point. If you are very active, you might need much more."* He also said, *"Children need a lot of protein. If you have a child who is growing, you might have 2X to 5X this amount: 2.4 g/kg (1.2 g/lb) or more".*

Eating such filling food will keep hunger away because it stabilizes your blood sugar and accordingly, your insulin level. Keeping a distance from addictive food (fast-acting carbohydrates) will support you in bringing balance back to your hormonal cycle of insulin, Leptin, Ghrelin, Glucagon, and others. This will help in decreasing the insulin and leptin resistance. As a bonus, it will let you reduce the amount of insulin taken if you are an insulin-dependent diabetic. Additionally, this also has the added benefit of making it easier to lose weight.

The second step is to be accustomed to skipping a meal daily until you are comfortable with that and then skip two meals until you feel just fine (You need to discuss this approach with your physician first). Eventually, you will be able to skip the three meals and fast for 24, 36 or 48 hours and perhaps even more if you want to. I have fasted for up to 4 days at one time with stable blood sugar and of course no ketoacidosis. However, I make sure my body has the proper level of basal insulin to close the loop of more production of ketones if any.

During fasting, you can drink water and any hot or cold non-caloric beverages. Experts advise you to take in some natural

Himalayan and Potassium salts to help manage electrolytes on longer fasts. I also take magnesium glycinate and apple cider vinegar. Again, please educate yourself on this topic, acclimate slowly, and consult with your physician before attempting extended fasting, especially if you are insulin-dependent with less experience dealing with external insulin. After a while, fasting will grant you a sense of well-being and will help you lose weight if this is your goal. Of course, if you are T1 or T2 diabetic you need to reduce your insulin or medicine accordingly in consultation with your physician.

The unlimited window of eating throughout the day does not allow our bodies a break. As a result, the processes of fat burning, restoration and repair could not be launched.

Our fast-paced lives, the food socialization, the easy access to meals, the business-oriented guidelines, and the food overconsumption are major problems of our modern societies. They leave us vulnerable to many metabolic and cognitive diseases along with their harmful consequences.

Chapter 7: Fasting and our smart Bodies

"A little starvation can really do more for the average sick man than can the best medicines and the best doctors."
Mark Twain

M ost diet programs work only for a while, it is likely that the body will hinder your progress and take you back to the square number one. Our bodies are well trained to protect us, according to its own understanding of protection. The Hypothalamus controls many crucial functions in our bodies. One of them is to keep a weight set point, so if you try to go below the set point, the hypothalamus does whatever it can to slow down or halt the whole weight loss process. It can launch hunger, regulate hormones, slow down your metabolism, make leptin receptors resistant to leptin or regulate your emotional responses to food. This is why, when starting a diet, many people lose weight first couple of weeks and find it hard to keep the weight off. They are out of the set point range thus the body is fighting back.

Let's say your body requires 2000 calories per day to survive but you are consuming around 1000 calories in an attempt to lose weight. With this amount of calories reduction, the **first thing your body will do** is to reduce the energy expenditure by reducing your metabolism. So, if you usually spend 800 calories while sleeping (a rough estimate) necessary for your organs to operate, your body will reduce its needs to 500 calories for example. One of the tools your body does to fight back the weight loss is making you leptin resistant. Leptin resistant people spend fewer calories compared to leptin's sensitive people, either during the sleeping time or while doing any similar activity! In other words, leptin resistance reduces your energy expenditure.[15]

In addition, a person who lost 10% of his body weight, his energy expenditure will be dropped by around 20%. This happens because when losing fat, the leptin production is reduced and the brain will not get the full message to keep the energy expenditure as it is. In the words of Dr. Sharma *"A 200 lb person, who loses 40 lbs burns about 20% fewer calories than someone who is 160 lbs but has never been obese. On top of this, the formerly-obese person experiences hunger, cold intolerance, other behavioral and metabolic changes that make sustaining this lower body weight difficult."*[16]

In fact, your body (Hypothalamus) has many tricks to use when it comes to saving you extra energy:

- It may make you lazy.
- It may increase your appetite.
- It may reduce your heart rate.
- It may reduce your leptin sensitivity so that your brain couldn't see your full fat reserves and as a result send a message to slow metabolism instead of the contrary.

The upshot is: when you reduce food intake, your body does everything possible to save you more energy; thinking you are deprived or in need of such energy because your incoming energy is less than what your brain thinks it is required to keep you alert and alive.

How are our bodies respond to fasting?

Knowing how smart our bodies are, I always asked myself this question: What about fasting? Will the body still have the same attitude while fasting? Will the brain hinder the weight loss efforts, expected by fasting, just as it does with calorie reduction diets?

I did not have a real answer to this question until I extensively searched the topic. In his Book <u>Complete guide to fasting</u>, Dr. Jason Fung said that fasting leads to secretion of Adrenaline, passing the hour 24 of fasting and by the hour 48 of fasting; the metabolism rate is raised by 3.6%. Ditto, the metabolic rate increases with great 14% and the resting expenditure increased by 12% when fasting for full four days.[1718] Unlike any calories reduction systems where the metabolic rate slows down in direct proportion with calories reduction. Some people might think this is controversial because people tend to eat more after fasting than the norms. I definitely respect this opinion but, again, I am a result-oriented person and my experience with fasting or refeeding was just amazing. I actually eat less after fasting. For some reason fasting partially blocks my appetite and I find myself not able to eat much after fasting.

It seems that with prolonged fasting, the body reaches a point that it has to start utilizing its own stored energy otherwise the vital functions will shut down. Doing that is a continuation of being a smart body. So why this is not happening when we eat little (reduce calories)? Perhaps the body still senses there is some energy coming in, so it still wants to make use of the incoming energy the optimum way possible. Therefore, the body tries to match its own needs by utilizing whatever energy admitted to it and, in the meantime, postpones using the stored energy (your fat guts) later. I am just thinking rational here.

During prolonged fasting, the body becomes even smarter by increasing your metabolism and burning more fat for fuel.[19] By doing so, it actually gives you extra energy (strength) to enable you to start moving and searching harder for food. It makes a great sense, isn't it? However, this leads us to another question. Whence the body will get this extra energy while there is no food eaten? The simple answer is, by utilizing the stored fat. The body gets the message that there is enough energy available to be utilized and starts to raise your metabolism so you can go out and start hunting your food.

Fasting for 24 hrs or more, varies from one to another, leads to release ketones as substitute energy to glucose. Obviously, this happens because of the absence of insulin when you fast. There is no consumed food to raise your insulin level, hence your body has no choice but to search for the stored energy (fat) and start burning it instead of glucose. When you fast, you are in a fat burning mode. You are not in fat storage mode anymore.

Do we lose muscles while fasting

There is a famous assertion says that fasting or prolonged fasting, in specific, burns your muscles for energy instead of fat! Dr. Fung mentioned that this is too dummy to be done with such a smart machine like your body. Burning the stand-by energy (glycogen), fat, when food is scarce, is a natural mechanism. Therefore, why will the smart body leave the stored fat untouched (which meant to be used in these circumstances) and starts decomposing our muscles for energy?![20] The body knows that we need those muscles to obtain the required food. Those old days in history, the one method allowed human to get food, is to hunt. In other words "to put efforts". If the body goes dormant, it means; it is a stupid body and that isn't true. Still, there are no constants in science as every opinion could be partially right or wrong, but this opinion here makes a lot of sense to me.

Human growth hormone (HGH) is one of the major hormones that motivates weight loss through burning fat. When we get older, our bodies reduce the production of HGH. One of the HGH's functions is to guard our muscles' mass and bones density, as HGH is designed to build not to destroy.

Scientists found that one of the most potent stimuli for HGH production is prolonged fasting. A 1992 study found a fivefold increase in growth hormone after two days of fasting.[21] Another study found that three days of fasting causes HGH levels to increase by over 300% and after forty days of religious fasting, HGH increases by a huge 1,250% (from 0.73 ng/ml to 9.86 ng/ml).[22] This is alone makes you understand the importance of fasting in fat weight loss without muscles mass loss.[23]

In brief, long-term studies of intermittent fasting prove that a fasting strategy is better than low calorie diets at preserving lean mass percentage compared to caloric restriction due to the effect of the elevated growth hormone caused by fasting.[24][25] Also, fasting causes Noradrenalin to rise, keeping metabolism high in diet-induced obese male mice.[26]

T1 diabetic has to avoid diabetes ketoacidosis (DKA), while fasting, by keeping blood sugar in the normal range and continuing their basal insulin. Intermittent Fasting with controlled blood sugar and with a proper level of basal insulin in the body will only lead to nutritional ketosis, not to DKA. This concept is commonly misunderstood by many medical professionals. Again, a person with T1 and T2 diabetes should consult his/her physician before fasting for medication adjustment.

Many of us have never experienced nutritional ketosis, as we leave no room and time for utilizing our stored fat. In fact, our bodies have become fat storing machines as we live in a state of continuous feeding. When we are in this state, we are absolutely going against our manufacture's catalog. We are not programmed to have food available all the time. We must search, plant and hunt it.

Prophet Mohamed (peace be upon him) said *"No man fills a container worse than his stomach. A few morsels that keep his back upright are sufficient for him. If he has to, then he should keep one-third for food, one-third for drinking and one-third for his breathing."* The true wisdom of this Hadeeth (quote) sums it up all. You should never fill up your stomach to the maximum extent; otherwise, it will influence your health negatively. You only need a little food to enable you to move around, be active and take care of your daily chores. The rest is waste.

Fasting provides a clear mind and body. Fasting is a natural state we faced in our daily lives, over and over in history, when food was scarce. Fasting improves our health as it cleanses our bodies from within. It allows the recycle of malignant, weak and dead cells through Apoptosis and Autophagy processes. Fasting improves insulin sensitivity and makes you lose excess weight with no money spent. Above all, it makes normalizing blood sugar a piece of cake.

A couple a week of intermittent fasting up to 24 hours a day helped me to control my blood sugar, reduce my bolus insulin to zero, during fasting, reduce my basal about 30%, prevent the food cravings and maintain my weight perfectly.

Chapter 8: The Choice

"The three rules for getting control of your diet. Rule 1. If you're OK, you're OK. Rule 2. If you want to lose weight: Don't eat. If you have to eat, don't eat carbs. If you have to eat carbs, eat low-glycemic index carbs. Rule 3. If you have diabetes or metabolic syndrome, carbohydrate restriction is the "default" approach, that is, the one to try first."
Richard David Feinman

S uzan stared away trying not to recall that drastic day, as it fills her with bitter memories. The day she discovered her son Adam had type one diabetes twenty years ago. He was five years old at the time. Adam was admitted to the hospital after losing, unexplainably, 6 lb of his weight along with many symptoms like thirst and frequent urination. He was then diagnosed with T1 diabetes and spent about one week in the hospital attempting to lower his blood sugar and his high ketones level resulting from diabetic ketoacidosis.

Susan was given a little booklet at the hospital to learn about diabetes control basics. This booklet led her to read many other books about diabetes management and nutrition. In twenty years, Suzan was fully responsible for Adam's blood sugar management.

It was not hard for her to learn that blood sugar levels above normal range are the real cause of all complications not diabetes itself, as it is mistakenly known to many people with diabetes.

She realized the importance of strict normalization of Adam's blood sugar otherwise; he might get many painful complications within 10 years in the most optimistic scenario. She centralized her life around controlling Adam's blood sugar all the time. Her ultimate dream was to see him a healthy young man. All these years, she kept on visualizing him sitting head up, healthy and happy beside his bride at his marriage ceremony.

Twenty years passed and here he is, sitting right there in front of her exhausted eyes with his beautiful bride. He is a strong and healthy young man who did not lose a limb, kidney or a nerve to diabetes because of his brave and smart mother.

Certainly, many friends and family members blamed her for being so assertive about Adam's food choices. She was also blamed for getting herself and the rest of the family all centered on controlling his blood sugar. She never settled for something less than normal blood sugar. Nevertheless, she always kept in her mind the beautiful quote of the legendary Dr. Richard Bernstein *"If you want to control your blood sugar you must know about diabetes just like your physician does."* Suzan printed this eternal quote in many copies. She hung it everywhere her eyes would touch upon: the mirror, the fridge, the closet, the car, and even her workstation. All the family could read it tens of times daily until it became a way of living for them. Suzan only changed two words in the quote to be *"If you want to control your blood sugar, you must know about diabetes more than your physician does"*

Time passed like a rocket and here she is; thinking about the long journey with diabetes while celebrating the day she always dreamed of "Adam's wedding".

Swiftly, she was brought from the past to the present moment by a whispering voice from behind. A voice she knew very well, saying, "Congratulations Suzan, it seems you will be a grandmother soon."

It was her close friend Sara. She has known Sara for 20 years. Unfortunately, they had not seen each other in the past 5 years as Sara and her family had moved to another state for work.

Sara came to attend the wedding with her son Sammy who is a dear friend of Adam as well. Sammy was diagnosed with T1 diabetes almost at the same time as Adam. Coincidentally, both families were introduced to each other at the same hospital, where both Adam and Sammy received the initial T1 diabetes treatment.

Sara always blamed Suzan, quietly, being so fanatic and strict about Adam's blood sugar control. She particularly resented that Suzan had prohibited some popular foods from entering her house since Adam was diagnosed. Suzan excluded starches, juices, sugar, potatoes, and wheat because she learned that the wrong dietary choices were doing severe harm to people with diabetes by keeping their blood sugar always out of control. She did not only learn this but she examined it by monitoring Adam's unstable BS profile when eating such food.

Suzan knew with a lot of reading along with day-to-day experience that Adam could never be able to control his blood sugar eating this kind of food. Therefore, she started to learn low carb's cooking and to discover all possible alternatives to the prohibited food. Her goal was to enable Adam to stick to the low carbohydrate way of eating without feeling deprived of anything. In the meantime, Sara adopted the idea of letting Sammy ate whatever he wanted and injected insulin (bolus) for it. Her famous statement was "let him eat like his peers and friends, so he will be mentally fine and doesn't feel deprived." Of course, this attitude caused continuous high blood sugar and various complications to Sammy that, unfortunately, revealed themselves badly in the future.

They sat together chatting about the wedding, the bride dress, and many bitter and sweet memories. They talked about how fast time passed and how babies are getting married now. Suddenly Sammy stood up and headed directly to congratulate his dear friend Adam. Suzan noticed there was a little limp in Sammy's walk. She asked Sara, "Is Sammy Limping?!"

Sadly, Sara paused for about 10 seconds and said with tears in her eyes, "I deeply wished I had listened to your advice regarding Sammy's diabetes management. Sammy injured his foot a year ago and he wasn't able to feel the wound because of his severe foot neuropathy. To make a long story short, it led to his foot amputation," Sara continued saying, "*Your words still ring in my ears: 'The real control of the blood sugar of our diabetic sons is a choice and every choice has its own consequences'.*"

Chapter 9: The three meals myth

"If you cannot control your hunger and appetite, good luck managing your blood chemistry, metabolism, waistline, and, in the bigger picture, the prospect of crippling your brain."
Dr. David Perlmutter.

O besity becomes a phenomenon that cannot be overlooked. I invite you to look closer to the sizes of the people around and you will definitely realize the severity of the problem. Most of us cannot run, jog or even walk briskly because of the accumulated fat surrounds our bodies and hinder our mobility. What makes it even worse is that obesity goes side by side with type 2 diabetes. Statistics show that for every five people with T2 diabetes, four of them are overweight.[27]

According to the National Institute of Diabetes and Digestive and Kidney Diseases (NIDDK), two out of every three adults are overweight, one out of every three adults is obese and one adult out of every 13 is extremely obese. The most concerning, however, is the alarming increase in the number of children with obesity. One-third of kids between the ages of 9 to 16 are overweight and one in 16 children and adolescents ages 2 to 19 is considered obese.[28] No wonder the number of kids diagnosed with T2 diabetes is escalating. An Indonesian study shows that the prevalence of type 2 diabetes in children and adolescents has increased globally over the past 2 decades. The study mentioned *"metabolic syndrome, including obesity and overweight at a young age, increases the occurrence of T2D"*[29]

In my diabetes management FB page, I sadly receive many messages from parents of teenagers that have been diagnosed with T2 diabetes. When I ask about the kids' weight, the answers were 99% of them are overweight. I always advise them to seek medical and nutritional advice to control the weight and improve the dietary habits and this usually brings fruitful results on reversing their early T2 diagnosis. To visualize the severity of the problem, you need to know that T2 diabetes diagnosis was primarily seen in people above 30 years old. Twenty years ago, it was rare that children or adolescents got diagnosed with T2 diabetes.

Poor dietary habits drive obesity, which plays a big role in causing T2 diabetes among children. Development of T2 diabetes at such a young age appears to compound the adverse effect of the disease. The outcomes on the health of those unfortunate kids are exponential.

I watched one of the widely shared videos on FB showing New York City recorded back in 1911. This video shows many daily life scenes in 1911. I tried to pinpoint one fat person in the video, but I failed. It was just unbelievable. Please check the video here https://bit.ly/2qxwC8a

As we all know, obesity is the fastest highway to many diseases such as diabetes, coronary heart diseases, high blood pressure, strokes, joints pain, Alzheimer, and others. Dr. William Davis in his book <u>Wheat Belly</u> said that the main culprit for obesity in our world is modern wheat. He elaborated about the effect of the starch ingredient in wheat known as "Amylopectin A".

Dr. Davis said it very well, *"Wheat triggers a cycle of insulin-driven satiety and hunger, paralleled by the ups and down euphoria and withdrawal, distortions of neurological function, and addictive effects, all leading to fat deposition. The extreme of blood sugar and insulin are responsible for the growth of fat specifically in the visceral organs.*

Experienced over and over again, visceral fat accumulates creating a fat liver, two fat kidneys, a fat pancreas, a fat large and small intestines, as well as its familiar surface manifestation, a wheat belly."[30]

One of the major components of modern wheat is a protein called gluten, which has a huge adverse influence on our bodies and brains. Although gluten is a real problem, this book is not to discuss it. If you wish to learn more about it, I recommend you read Dr. William Davis's book along with Dr. David Perlmutter book Grain Brain.

Simply put, the more you consume food that rapidly converts to glucose such as wheat, sugar, and starches, the more you store fat and become unable to burn it later if you still eat the same kind of food. **The more fast-acting carb foods → More Glucose in bloodstream → more insulin secreted → Overweight or Obesity → insulin resistance → high possibility of diagnosed with T2 diabetes.**

So the major two problems extensively contribute in the prevalence of both obesity and T2 diabetes, in my opinion, are that *we eat the wrong food and that we eat too much of it* at the same time. In other words, we eat *Sugar and starches* and we *eat A LOT* of them. So, here comes the crucial questions: Do we really need to eat three meals a day? The short answer is no.

The three meals per day myth,

Let's assume your weight is 100 KG including 30 KG of fat. Each gram of fat can generate about 9 calories when burned as energy. In other words, you carry around 270,000 calories worth of unused energy stored in your body.

For the sake of argument, let's assume your body needs around 2000 calories per day to perform well. In This case, mathematically, the unused stored fat in your body will be sufficient for you to live 135 days. Imagine the fat storage mechanism meant to feed you when food is scarce is not in service anymore. Therefore, we are in a state of storage only. You keep on storing fat but never allow it to be utilized because you are in a constant feeding condition (The three meals and snacks). There is no chance for the stored fat to be burned in place of the dominant fuel, glucose.

Amazingly, the longest fasting trial in our modern history was back in 1966 by a 27 years old male who fasted for 382 days under the supervision of Scotland University. He started his fasting weighed 456 lb (207 kg) and ended it up weighing 180 lb (82 kg). He lost a total weight of 276 lb (125 kg). During his fasting, he was given water, vitamin supplements, potassium, and yeast.[31]

Of course, I am not suggesting you fast for 382 days, but what I am arguing about here is that we can survive, even during such extreme starvation state, assuming we have the right medical supervision, water, and some supplements, and needed stored fat. Because, in fact, stored fat is unused energy.

Actually, the type of food (fast-acting carbs) we excessively eat causes dependency on the easy fuel (glucose) and neglect the other source of fuel that is already stored as fat in our bodies.

By gulping more of wheat, rice, sugar, and pasta, we push the pancreas to secrete more insulin to cover the extra glucose eaten and this initiates the storage of the excess glucose as glycogen in the liver and muscles. Then the remaining glucose, combined with fatty acids, will be stored as triglyceride (FAT). Insulin is a fat hormone. insulin induces fat cells to store more fat via stimulating an enzyme called Lipoprotein lipase (LPL) which open the way from outside-in to fat cell to admit three fatty acids molecules and one glucose molecule to form Triglyceride (the dense stored form of fat).

At the meantime, Insulin deactivates another enzyme called High Sensitive Lipase (HSL) located inside fat cells. HSL is responsible for the disassembly of TG again to its components of fatty acids and glucose. The fatty acids are released into the bloodstream to be burned as a clean fuel to operate our bodies in the absence of enough glucose.

The three meals a day is not something you must do, it is just a ritual we get used to. Have you ever recollect a day in your life you were so busy, so you run to work without breakfast. Then you were hooked up in many activities and meetings during the day. Then back home around 7 pm, got your dinner, watched some TV, and slept. Had you noticed the whole day passed by with a single meal and some cups of tea and coffee? **Do you remember what happens to you that day?**

- Did you feel weak?
- Did you faint?
- Did you die!
- Did you suffer any kind of malnutrition?
- Did your performance at work was badly influenced?

In fact, nothing happens at all. Perhaps you felt better that day with a clearer mind and lighter body than other days where you ate five meals on them. Isn't it?

Let go of your sacred morning meal

When I began to reduce my food intake, I found that I could nicely get away with a breakfast of one egg or two. I was no longer in need of the famous TV breakfast of milk, orange juice, cereals, cheese, beans, a hero, falafel or whatever I used to devour on my sacred morning meal. With a bit more effort and understanding, I found out that I was in no need breakfast at all. In fact, I never bought the myth of "breakfast is the most important meal of the day." I am a firm believer of what Dr. Fung said *"Breakfast: the most important meal to skip."* It is just a break-fast, and I do not want to break my fast in the morning. I am totally fine with that.

Skipping breakfast helped me deal with dawn phenomenon as an insulin-dependent diabetic. The dawn phenomenon (DP) is when blood sugar gets elevated early morning and there is not enough insulin to cover it in people with T1 diabetes or less insulin (insulin resistance) to cover it in T2 diabetes. My DP is severe when my liver is full of glycogen. Every day when I wake up I need to inject three or four units of fast insulin even if my BS is OK, except if I was fasting for 36 hours or more.

Skipping breakfast also led me to 19 hours of fasting, from 8 pm the night before to 3 pm the same day. Doing this rests my mind, body and digestion system. It also helped me control my blood sugar and maintain my weight. Did I feel weak doing this? Not at all, I felt more energetic indeed. I only add some Himalayan and potassium salt along with magnesium glycinate.

To appreciate food and know the difference between abundance and scarcity of food, I want you to imagine the following. Back 10,000 years ago in the Savanah and before the Era of food abundance, getting your daily food depended primarily on four factors: Skills, efforts, fitness, and luck. Therefore, you always have one of the four scenarios happen all the time:

1. If you put forth efforts, you are lucky and skilful but you are not fit, you are not able to run, climb or swim - Imaginably, you will end up with no food.
2. If you are Skilful, fit and put forth required efforts but have no luck, you will still have the same results of no food.
3. If you are fit, put the required efforts and lucky but not skilful, again, there will be no food as well.
4. Finally, if you are lucky, fit and skilful but not willing to put efforts, then you will sleep hungry again this night.

Being able to keep your catch, until you get back to your cave for your family, purely depends on luck. Bad luck can show itself in a form of hungry predator walking past who also in search for his lunch. If your luck is terrible, that predator will pinpoint you like a big meal! If that happens, then you will lose it all: your catch and your life! You will see this in Khamis story later in an upcoming chapter.

Considering all these factors along with food scarcity, most likely you will end up with a meal every couple of days. You may eat a portion of it and keep the rest until tomorrow. However, if the catch was huge, you and your tribe will feast. This is fine because your thrifty genes will jump in and do their instinctual job of storing the extra food as body fat, which will be used in the next couple of days when food is scarce again. There was no possibility of keeping the extra weight or fat because of the ongoing food scarcity.

Therefore, in my opinion, one of the simplest solutions to help in controlling blood sugar, to lose weight and to improve insulin resistance is to forget about the myth of the necessity for three meals a day. Additionally, we need to imitate our ancestors and pretend there is not plenty of food ready all the time. In short, we need to tolerate a little raucousness and asceticism. By doing so, we will allow our stored fat to melt away and reverse any possible symptoms of T2 diabetes that might show up already.

Therefore, if you are T2 diabetic, pre-diabetic, overweight or obese, I suggest the following:

First:

Get rid of the idea of eating all the time, what I called in my other book, written in Arabic (In Love, Life and Open Buffet), The Open Buffet Syndrome (OBS). Remove the OBS from your brain (mentally) and then from your house (physically). Do not have a house full of food all the time. Decide that there are days you are not lucky in hunting and food is scarce. Then, you may be lucky and catch a gazelle and feast or you may catch a little rabbit that allows you only one small meal for the next three days.

Second:

Eat dinner early around 7 pm and skip breakfast the next day. Then eat lunch at 3 pm. This way you have fasted for almost 20 hours. Then after a couple of days, skip both breakfast and lunch altogether and eat at 7 pm again. This way you have almost fasted 24 hours. Soon, your meal will automatically shrink. Of course, while fasting, you can drink and get the required natural sea salt or Himalayan salt, magnesium, and potassium. You definitely need to consult your physician and please read Dr. Fung's book The

<u>Complete Guide To Fasting</u>. It is a great source of information about fasting techniques.

If you have diabetes and you do this, you will control your blood sugar. If you are overweight, you will lose weight without feeling hungry all the time. You will also have better odds against T2 diabetes, insulin resistance, coronary heart diseases, high blood pressure, stroke, digestion issues, and cognitive diseases.

Fasting will also help in the prevention of Cancer. Please read Dr. Thomas Seyfried book <u>Cancer as a Metabolic Disease</u> for more information on this topic.

Chapter 10: Fasting and the fate of Khamis

"We are wired for feast and famine, not feast, feast, feast."
Dr. Jason Fung.

G et a cup of coffee, relax and visualize with me, you went back in history. You live in a jungle about 20,000 years ago. There were no villas, buildings, luxury homes, penthouse or whatever. You got no choice but to live in a hidden cave out there in nowhere. You have a non-fatty, masculine and flexible body. Everything you have to get in life is linked to your ability to move, run, walk, climb or swim.

Unfortunately, this week you were not lucky hunting something to eat. The last meal you and your family ate was almost ninety-six hours ago. Back in those days, there was no other way you can get a meal rather than hunting?" There was no place, where you can buy ready hunted food. No hypermarket, No grocery stores, no restaurants, no fridges, no deep freezers, no stored food and of course, no delivery. If you want to eat you have to hunt, it is that simple.

So, to feed your family, you must come out of your cave, leave your stony couch and repeatedly try to catch something to eat because your kids are starving already. Therefore, you decided to double your hunting force and get some help by inviting your neighbor "Khamis" to go hunt with you. Khamis lives about two kilometers away from you. No WhatsApp or messenger to text him, no mobile or landline phones. You have to walk over two kilometers to his cave and get him to go out hunting with you. Khamis and his family were about 96 hours without food as well.

You arrived there at the foothill and called Khamis with maximum voice. The eco helped you to transmit your calling to Khamis. Khamis came down running with his belly and double chin dancing right and left, while going down the hill from his cave to you. Yes, unlike you, Khamis was chubby.

Together, you looked around for something to hunt, any rabbit, gazelle, bird, or snake - anything. Hours passed but no luck, sunset is around the corner and still no catch. Now you both are starving and have no more energy to spend running behind this and that. Therefore, you called it off for the day before darkness covers everything. It, sadly, seems the 96 hours of fasting will be dragged to 120 hours for you, Khamis and both families.

Suddenly, on the way back to caves, a huge hungry tiger was also out to hunt, and the imminent danger leaves you and Khamis in big mental labyrinth! You either have to fight or flight and of course, with such a beast, flight is the only sane action you both can take. Therefore, you and Khamis fled as fast as you can. Now, fitness here is an indispensable trait and without it, you are a dinner instead of a hunter. In one sad moment, Khamis did not make it and the hungry tiger caught him. In fact, his extra fat will satisfy the predator for three more days. Sadly, Khamis is gone and became a memory in a minute. Actually, the tiger devoured Khamis because he could not run faster.

One of the main pillars to stay alive at that time in history was to be fit, fast and sharp. Being fat was fatal, unlike nowadays where you can be fat and no carnivores will attack you or eat you alive. However, if you contemplate a little deeper, you will figure out that there are many predators disguising in different shapes in contemporary time.

Those modern predators still attack both fit and unfit human but it prefers to attack the unfit and the overweight, the smoker, and the unhealthy food eater. Their names are not Tigers, Lions, hyenas, crocodiles, or wolves. They have different modern names we all know very well. Names like diabetes, Obesity, high blood pressure, heart diseases, stroke, Alzheimer, etc.

Every five persons get T2 diabetes, four of them are overweight! This doesn't say "the only reason to get T2 diabetes is being overweight or obese," but it says, "being overweight is one of the major reasons can get you T2 diabetes easily." In fact, the best action to be taken right after been diagnosed with T2 diabetes is to lose weight and that itself improves a lot the condition and almost reverse it all.

Let me give you an example about me as a LADA diabetic, which is exactly like being T1 Diabetic with more insulin resistance. A LADA diabetic injects insulin in form of basal insulin once or twice every 24 hours depends on the type of insulin and injects bolus insulin with food. During my journey with diabetes I found out if I lose 5% of my weight, I reduce my basal about 10% and if I lose 10% of my weight; I reduce basal with about 20% of my total daily basal. Not only this, but my insulin sensitivity improves when I lose weight, which allows me to use less bolus insulin with the same amount of carbohydrates eaten. In general, I eat about 30 grams per day or less.

Those days of Khamis and you were the norms in our history. At that time, the one and only simple dominant rule of feeding was: **"You find food you feast; you do not find food you fast until you find food"**. It is that simple. You may have three meals a day, then two weeks without even a bite of food. It is mandatory fasting. Well, no one in those days talked about the necessity of specific daily calories, macros or vitamins that must be consumed. Eating was driven by the availability of food. That is it.

The time you have some extra food, you eat and store unneeded energy as fat around your organs, which your body will use it naturally when food is scarce. For this reason, you are always in between feeding state and nutritional ketosis (NK) state. In NK, you synthesize your body fat and use it as a substitute source of energy, so you will not die.

To shift your paradigm about continuous feeding state, assume you are there with Khamis and act accordingly. You just assume you not supposed to have shelves packed with ready, processed food full of artificial preservative. You need to assume you have no extra food to store for the next meal and live accordingly. It was only when I began to squeeze two to three days of fasting in my week, my insulin sensitivity improved a lot along with positive maintenance of my weight, which was horrible to control while injecting much insulin.

Our ancestors did not get the honey in jars. If they wanted to eat honey, they must climb the trees and fight the bees for a lick or two. Food never meant to be found in abundance just like the case with us now. Because of such abundance, we become in a continuous feeding state and as a result in a continuous illness state as well.

Chapter 11: How did I get my HbA1c from 10 to 5

"The typical response from people when I tell them I am diabetic is, 'Oh, I'm sorry to hear that.' You know, I am not. I am a better athlete because of diabetes rather than despite it. I am more aware of my training, my fitness and more aware of nutrition. I am more proactive about my health."

Charlie Kimball

S ince I was diagnosed back in 2003 and for nearly eight years, my HbA1c was between 8% to 11% all the time. As advised, I was following a low fat, medium protein, and high Wholewheat carbohydrates diet. I never had real control over my blood sugar during those eight years. The learning journey started by the end of 2010 onwards. So let me head directly to the point. What exactly I had done and still do, to control my blood sugar and to reduce my HbA1c from 10% to 5.5%? What measures did I take to gain the control back? I will answer these questions through the following topics. Each topic contributed to achieving normal blood sugar. Let's start.

Knowledge is power

Yes, knowledge is power. I am talking about the knowledge that brings results when applied. The knowledge that makes a positive difference in one's life. From 2011 onwards, I learned not to follow blindly when it comes to BS control. If something I read convinces me, I apply it to myself and judge it by my blood sugar readings. I consider diabetes control is a self-evident matter. In other words, I can notice whether I am in control by just monitoring my blood sugar. I can feel the onset of complications because of uncontrolled blood sugar. I can see the immediate effect of any kind of food on my BS and energy level. And, I can differentiate easily between the effect of sugar and starches on my BS compared to the effect of meat, healthy fat or non-starchy vegetables.

In the beginning of 2010, I started to look for the right books written by knowledgeable people in diabetes management and nutrition. I began with three books:

- Dr. Bernstein's Diabetes Solution by Dr. Richard K. Bernstein.
- Think Like A Pancreas by Gary Scheiner.
- Blood Sugar 101, What They Don't Tell You About Diabetes by Jenny Ruhl.

With these three books, I learned how to master many techniques, which in turn helped me in achieving normal blood sugar, as I will explain later.

What are the values of normal blood sugar

In order for me to achieve normal BS, I needed to observe what was happening with my BS profile in the twenty-four hours. What kind of foods raises my blood sugar and what don't? "Seeing is believing". So, I began measuring my BS about 8 to 10 times a day to understand the effect of various types of food on my BS. This alone confirmed the huge negative effect of fast-acting carbohydrates on my blood sugar and this is what Dr. Bernstein preaches about all the time.

After years of uncontrolled BS, I badly wanted to learn about the BS target I needed to follow. By default, physicians put us on ADA BS target. When this did not work with me for years, I thought, perhaps I needed to follow the target of the American Association of Clinical Endocrinologists (AACE), which is lesser than the ADA BS target. However, when I knew the normal BS level, I rejected the AACE target.

The hard question I asked myself repeatedly at that time was: even if I knew the normal blood sugar target, can I achieve it? When I asked this question to many of the physicians I dealt with, the answer was always, I can never be able to achieve normal blood sugar because I am a diabetic.

As I am writing this now, it reminded me of what happened with Dr. Bernstein back in 1972, when he requested a computer search of the scientific literature from the local medical library. He wanted to know about the possibility of reversing diabetes complications as he was suffering from many of them. When he received the report, he discovered that diabetes complications could be prevented and even reversed in animals by normalizing blood sugar. Dr. Bernstein said in his book "*Excited by my discovery, I showed this report to my physician, who was not impressed. 'Animal aren't humans,' he said, and besides, 'it's impossible to normalize human blood sugar.' Since I had been trained as an engineer, not as a physician, I knew nothing of such impossibilities, and since I was desperate, I had no choice but to pretend I was an animal.*"[32]

My physician had the same opinion of Dr. Bernstein's physician regarding normal BS achievement. As I said, he advised me to follow the ADA BS target for years, which is way far from normal BS and following it caused me many complications. That was, of course, before I read to Dr. Bernstein. After all the suffering with the uncontrolled blood sugar and after reading Dr. Bernstein's book, I finally opted for the normal blood sugar.

However, the term "normal blood sugar" has been highly disputed. It seems everyone has a different reference for normal blood sugar. This propelled me to research this subject extensively and I even measured the blood sugar of many of my non-diabetic friends and close family. I greatly needed to understand what normal blood sugar numbers really are!

In his book, Dr. Bernstein said that the normal BS is around **83 mg/dl** most of the time. By digging a bit more, I stumbled on a great article by Jenny Ruhl (it is also written in her book, blood sugar 101) about the real values of normal blood sugar. In her article,[33] Jenny mentioned the famous study of Prof. J.S. Christiansen who presented his valuable study back in September 2006 in the major annual European Diabetes Conference.

In his study, Prof. Christiansen used CGM and high carb food to find out the normal blood sugar ranges for normal non-diabetic subjects. His results can be concluded as follows: normal blood sugar was 125 mg/dl for a short period after a high carb meal. This reading was taken 45 minutes after eating, which considered a blood sugar peak after a starchy meal. Then Blood sugar drops to under 100 mg/dl by 75 minutes after eating and stays around 85 mg/dl by one hour and forty-five minutes after eating. While fasting blood sugar remains around low 80s mg/dl all night long.[34]

Considering all the above data, I concluded that my blood sugar target should be as follows,

- **Under 5.5% HbA1c.**
- **75 to 92 mg/dl fasting.**
- **Below 120 mg/dl, one hour after food.**
- **Below 100 mg/dl, two hours after food**.

The above numbers was my BS target since late 2010 until now. Frankly, I figured out that the only chance for me to reverse most of the diabetes complications and stop the deterioration of the non-reversible ones was to stick, long enough, to normal blood sugar. When I managed to keep my BS normal for a while, I was able to reverse my frozen shoulder complication and cystopathy issue as well. The diabetic cystopathy issue had given me a nightmarishly hard time for two years because of the similarity in symptoms with prostate issues. For your information, diabetic cystopathy is a chronic complication of diabetes with classic symptoms of decreased bladder sensation, increased bladder capacity, and impaired detrusor contractility.[35] Almost every urologist treated me as it was a prostate issue while it was not. Until one smart urologist figured it out but he did not tell me that normalizing BS could fix it. Luckily, after two years of normal BS, all symptoms started to improve dramatically, thanks to Dr. Bernstein.

The moral here is: It does not require a confirmation from anybody to realize that normal actions lead to normal reactions and abnormal actions lead to abnormal reactions. The same concept applies to blood sugar targets as well. So, please let no one convince you the abnormal BS range that ADA (or any other organization) wants you to follow is good for you. It is definitely not. There is nothing better to target, for PWD, than achieving normal blood sugar. And, if, for any reason, you do not trust the normal blood sugar target I mentioned above, please find five non-diabetic and healthy relatives or friends and ask them to measure their blood sugar fasting, one and two hours after food and you will confirm it by yourself!

The insulin choices and factors

Once I finished reading Dr. Bernstein book, I immediately deleted the pre-mixed insulin from my life. I substituted it with two types of insulin, the fast-acting insulin and long-acting one. In other words, I started the multiple daily injection system (MDI) about eight years ago. In brief, in MDI you inject fast or short-acting insulin (bolus) with every meal you eat (according to the carbohydrates and protein grams counts) and Basal insulin twice a day if it is Lantus or Tresiba and three times a day if it is Levemir as advised by Dr. Bernstein. Again, please follow whatever works with you and do not take any advice for granted. Search it, try it, ask your doctor about it and only stick to what brings you normal blood sugar.

For example, while Levemir works well with many, it does not work with me. Lantus gave me better results and Tresiba gave me the best results. With Levemir, I had to add about 40% extra units of my daily basal units compared to Lantus or Tresiba. It was like injecting insulin diluted with water.

Later I used Tresiba, once every 24 hours, and I was doing fine although Dr. Bernstein advised taking Tresiba twice a day. I agree that twice a day can work just fine for some people, but for me, once/24 hours was just enough. About four years ago, I started using the insulin pump. I usually switch back to MDI for three months every year to allow my skin to rest from the pump. Anyway I prefer the MDI over the pump, I like to be free.

The MDI or insulin pump approach granted me flexibility and confidence. It allowed me to adjust my bolus, basal and correction insulin units to exactly what I needed. Earlier I was injecting fixed daily dose of Pre-mixed insulin, as per my physician advice, and ate like an elephant to treat the frequent daily hypoglycemia and hyperglycemia caused by high fixed doses of injected insulin. It was a big mess! I know I mentioned this many times but again, never inject fixed doses of fast or short-acting insulin. Just inject according to carb count (protein as well) in your meal.

Insulin factors:

Knowing and mastering insulin factors is one of the most important tools that will make a difference in controlling your blood sugar. There are three main insulin factors you need to learn about:

1. **Insulin: carbs ratio (IC ratio)**

I initially estimated my IC ratio theoretically by using weight or by the total daily-injected insulin units (both basal and bolus) charts. Then I fine-tuned it by continuous measuring of my blood sugar two, three and four hours after eating until I confirmed my exact IC ratio. The process of identifying my IC ratio lasted about three weeks, and then I figured out that every unit of fast-acting insulin (FAI) covers four grams of carbohydrate. So, my IC ration = four.

2. **Correction factor (CF) or the so-called sensitivity factor**

The CF is the number of mg/dl of glucose in your bloodstream that can be lowered by one injected unit of fast-acting insulin. You can also calculate an approximate CF from the equation: **CF = 1800/ Number of total daily insulin (bolus and basal).** Then fine-tune it with BS measurements three to four after correction until you reach your target blood sugar reliably each time. The number 1800 could be between 1600 to 2200. As per John Walsh, the author of <u>Using Insulin,</u> you can use a number smaller than 1800 if your total basal dose represents less than 50% of your total daily insulin dose (TDD). You can also use a number higher than 1800, if your total basal represents more than 50% of your TDD.[36]

After a couple of BS corrections, you will easily figure out your exact CF. This will help you to keep your BS always in the normal range if it goes up. I only correct with FAI like Novolog, Apidra or Humalog. I never correct using short acting insulin (Humulin R or Actrapid) because it is not as fast as FAI in bringing BS down. When you first want to know your correction factor, make sure you do not suffer any of the following:

1. Sickness like cold and flu.
2. Having any infection.
3. Ketoacidosis.
4. Just finished long or intensive work out.
5. Extreme high blood sugar.[37] (I become insulin resistant when my BS is 170 mg/dl or above)

Number 1, 2, 3 and 5 will make you insulin resistant while number 4 will make you insulin sensitive. Therefore, if you correct your BS while having one of these conditions, the BS measurement after correction will not give an accurate indication for your real correction factor. Always choose a normal condition when you are on the initial process of knowing your CF.

My CF is 15, which means if my Blood Sugar is 170 mg/dl and I want to take it down to 80 mg/dl, my equation will be as follows:

Number of FAI units needed for BS correction = (BS needed to be corrected–Target BS to be achieved)/Correction Factor = (170–80)/CF = 90/15 = six units of fast-acting insulin.

CF is a unique personal number, i.e. CF of 15 is only for me while yours will be different. Of course, before blood sugar correction you should make sure there is no effective insulin in your blood. In other words, no Insulin On board (IOB). Otherwise, there will be double insulin effect on your blood sugar when injecting the correction dose. Or else you can calculate your IOB and correct if you think your BS really needs to be corrected.

3. Third is Insulin on Board (IOB)

IOB means how much FAI still remaining in your bloodstream after injecting it. If you are on an insulin pump, IOB is usually calculated for you. If you are on MDI and injecting FAI, you need to be familiar with the duration FAI remains active in your bloodstream and when the last dose was given. In general, FAI stays about three to four hours in your body differs from one to another. For example, Novorapid lasts three hours in my bloodstream. Therefore, if I inject six units, then after two hours there will be two units of IOB still active in my bloodstream. If I want to correct (lower) my blood sugar, I need to consider these two units as IOB. I need to subtract them from the correction dose unless I am sure the remaining two units of insulin will cover part of the food I ate two hours ago. In this case, I can ignore them.

The dilemma of Dawn Phenomenon (DP)

One of the major problems I have faced in my journey with diabetes was the dawn phenomenon. In T1 diabetes, the BG elevates, more or less, at 3 am, or when you arise in the morning. I realized that in order for me to achieve total control of BS, I must control the DP. Again, I used the wisdom of seeing is believing. I committed, for a month, to wake up at one, three and five am to measure my BS.

My BS rises to about 150 mg/dl by 3 am and reaches around 180 mg/dl by 6 am. This rise was happening every night even with low carbs WOE regardless when I injected the night basal or how good the BS number was before sleeping.

To make a long story short, I would like to mention that insulin pump solved this dilemma forever by almost doubling my basal needs from 12 am to 9 am and reduce it to less than half during late morning and afternoon. The final basal setting in my pump looks like this,

Time	Units
From 9 am to 12 pm	1.5 units/hour
From 12 pm to 7 pm	0.7 units/hour
From 7 pm to 12 am	1.45 units/hour
From 12 am to 3 am	1.8 units/hour
From 3 am to 9 am	1.95 units/hour

As you can see, my nighttime's basal need is almost triple what I require during the daytime due to the huge glucose dumping by my crazy liver, while sleeping.

One of the great tools that helped me in adjusting my insulin pump's basal units setting, especially overnight, was the Freestyle Libre. I used it for six months. It is an FGM (flash glucose monitoring). Some people say it is not a CGM but I believe the outcome is similar. Freestyle Libre measuring blood sugar in the interstitial fluid through a sensor inserted 5 mm under the skin. You get a reading of your BS, at your convenience, by flashing the freestyle Libre reader above the sensor. By using the Libre, I was able to precisely figure out my BS pattern overnight and tweaked the timing of both Tresiba and Humulin N (while in MDI) to get the optimum results possible. Undoubtedly, this made the pump basal setting so easy.

I always wanted to see what would happen when I reduce the stored glycogen in my liver. So, I fasted, multiple times, three days in series to see what is happening when I deplete, on purpose, most of my liver storage of glycogen. By the end of the third day of continuous food fasting, I noticed my basal needs, while sleeping, was reduced by 30% - 40% and my DP evaporated! I didn't need to inject the three units of FAI before my feet touch the ground when arising as I ritually do every day.

By dividing the basal insulin according to my hour-to-hour needs via the insulin pump, I was able to reduce my total daily basal needs from 41 units of Tresiba, while on MDI, to 33.75 of FAI units with the insulin pump. Despite this was a great advantage but I still prefer the freedom of MDI over the insulin pump. So, I had to find out a solution for the DP with MDI.

How I controlled DP with MDI

Initially, I injected Tresiba at 11 pm. Tresiba nearly has no peak, so it didn't solve the DP alone and the early morning rise continued. Therefore, I reduced my Tresiba by about four units and instead added five units of Humulin N (intermediate-acting insulin) with the Tresiba, right before my sleeping time (11 pm). This worked fine because Humulin N peaks, with me, in about 2.5 to 4 hours after injection and clears out the bloodstream in about 8 to 10 hrs. That peak helped me to conquer the gradual rise of BS that starts about 2 to 3 am. Now, my nights go peacefully and I can take as much break as I want from my insulin pump.

Another solution I also beat the DP by injecting Tresiba at 11 pm, as usual, and then wake up at 1 am and inject three units of Humulin R (short-acting insulin). Humulin R peaks with me in about 1.5 to 2 hours and clears out in about 4 to 6 hours. This also worked very well but the negative side was the wake up at the middle of my sleep to do it.

Matching insulin with carbohydrates.

Matching the timing of insulin injection with different types of foods is an important skill to control BS. It was necessary for me to learn when to inject FAI in related to the food I consume. For example, if I eat any food that slowly raises my blood sugar such as non-starchy vegetables, I inject the FAI five minutes before I eat or at eating time. I have found this timing works well with me. If I eat any fast-acting carbohydrates like bread or rice (rarely happens), I have to inject about 15 to 20 mins before food or else about 10 mins before I eat but with intramuscular injection (right in my deltoid muscle).

Remember everyone is different. You can experiment with timing by moving the shot up or back by 5 minutes to see if it matches up with your meal better. For example, if you are going a little bit high after a meal, but going up on the amount of insulin brings you too low later. Then, you stick with the lower amount of insulin and move it 5 minutes earlier. If this improves things but not to normal, then move it another 5 minutes earlier, until you reach your target. If your insulin acts too quickly (i.e. you have a low before your food kicks in), then you need to move the insulin injection 5 minutes later.

Dealing with protein

With MDI, I inject for protein 20 to 30 minutes after eating it or else, I use square bolus in my insulin pump if I wear it. As Dr. Bernstein said, you can consider that 35% of ingested meat protein value (not weight grams) in grams, as grams of glucose. Some people say it could reach 50% but I found the 35% is ok with me. For example, a 100 gm of beef contains around 20 grams of protein. Considering the 35% rule I mentioned, you could expect the effect of seven grams of glucose on your BS due to eating this piece of meat. In other words, we can say 7% of ingested meat protein by weight get converted to glucose. So, if the piece of ingested beef weighted 100 gm, 7% of it will be 7 grams of glucose to be considered.

In my case and many others I know, this only happens when eating protein with a very low carb meal. With type two diabetes, where beta cells still partially fine, the effect of eating protein on raising blood sugar can be neglected. Of course, the protein effect on blood sugar is slow, gradual and easy to deal with.

Does Protein convert to glucose?

There is a theory says protein is not converted to glucose. It induces glucagon to signal the liver in order to synthesize some of the stored glycogen and accordingly release some glucose into the bloodstream. This is the closest theory indeed. Another theory says, part of the protein is converted to glucose in very low carb diet through a process called gluconeogenesis. Either way, the outcome is the same; we need to consider the effect of some glucose when ingesting protein with very low carb WOE.

Food choices

It is worth repeating, you can never have normal blood sugar as a T1 or T2 diabetic if you follow a high carb diet. By saying so, I do not want you to think I am dogmatic or a tunnel vision thinker, not at all. You can still get relatively good numbers of BS eating moderately high carbs food but you will never get excellent numbers. Every person with diabetes knows this. In fact, the good numbers will not protect you from painful complications and consequences. So, what you really want to aim for, is the excellent BS numbers if you want to live peacefully with diabetes. This is my opinion and the opinion of any impartial person. I confirmed it for myself with my daily experience. Many other people with diabetes I know also confirmed it with ongoing personal experiences.

The first thing I did to obtain normal BS was to eliminate every food raises it. I eliminated sugar, fructose, high fructose corn syrup, sodas, juices (natural or unnatural), bread, pasta, rice, potatoes, all wheat products (white, whole wheat, everything), oats, almost all grains, starchy vegetables, and fruits except berries. Of course, I am human and sometimes I slip but I don't get dragged and I always get back to my WOE as fast as possible.

I started to love the good fat such as natural butter, eggs, olive oil, coconut oil, and avocado though I do not eat much fat unless it comes naturally with protein or naturally with other food like butter/eggs, salad/olive oil and beef with own fat. I also eat protein until satiety. Because protein is a filling and dense food, it is hard to overconsume it even if you try. Additionally, leafy vegetables became a big part of my daily meal (not meals) as well.

I learned that saturated fat is a good fat choice as long you don't exaggerate eating it or mix it with sugar or starches. Gary Taubes said in <u>Why We Get Fat</u>, *"In total, more than 70 percent of the fat in lard will improve your cholesterol profile compared with what would happen if you replace that lard with carbohydrates. The remaining 30 percent will raise LDL cholesterol (bad) but also raise HDL (good). In other words, and hard as this may be to believe, if you replace the carbohydrates in your diet with an equal quantity of lard, it will actually reduce your risk of having a heart attack. It will make you healthier. The same is true for red meat, bacon and eggs, and virtually any other animal product we might choose to eat instead of the carbohydrates that make us fat. (Butter is slight exception, because only half the fat will definitely improve your Cholesterol profile; the other half will raise LDL but also raise HDL)."*[38]

Before starting the low carb way of eating, you must consult with your physician and nutritionist, as you need to reduce both bolus and basal insulin if you are T1 or reduce medication if you are T2. When doing so, please choose a physician who believes in your approach.

This step, specifically, will show dramatic improvement in your BS numbers. It will get you so close to your normal BS range especially if you learn how to maneuver with your bolus insulin to match your meals. In fact, the majority of FAI you inject is used to cover those sugary and starchy foods. Therefore, when you adopt this WOE, you will reduce your FAI big time. Accordingly, you will minimize both Hyperglycemia and Hypoglycemia. Moreover, you will lose weight easily, as an added bonus.

Let me give you a quick example of how you will reduce your insulin needs when you start eating low carbs. Assume my lunch is a sandwich (100 grams of wheat) and couple slices of Gouda Cheese, lettuce and mayonnaise. A piece of bread weighs 100 grams has 50 grams of fast-acting carbohydrate in it. I need to inject 12 units of Novorapid if I eat it. However, if I discard the bread from my lunch and I eat the rest, I will inject zero insulin for it.

That is why one of the biggest mistakes many physicians do is to prescribe fixed doses of FAI (3 times a day) to people with T1 diabetes. As a result, the poor T1 guy spends all day long eating starches trying to cover those industrial fixed doses of FAI to avoid hypoglycemia and to resist persistent hunger caused by those fixed doses. Unfortunately, many physicians insist on this practice because they don't know any other alternatives!

Find a supporter

If I am to write from today to the end of my life about the support I got (and still get) from my wife, Rehab, I still can't be grateful enough to her. From day one, Rehab supported me in my journey with diabetes with every way possible. She was in the boat with me from day one without hesitation. She did not care whether the ocean is rough or calm. She just jumped in. She became an expert in low carbohydrates cooking. Miraculously, I still eat bread, tarts, cakes, pretzels, rice, pies, etc. all healthy low carb. She is a master of huge numbers of recipes that make me feel I did not give up any food at all. She eats low carb as well; she lost 10 kg of her weight as a result and reversed metabolic syndrome symptoms at very early stage. She learned every little detail of diabetes management. She can talk glycogen, Amylin, glucagon, leptin, IC ratio, IOB and more. You name it! I am so thankful to her beyond the words can express and I truly believe that my journey would have been failure without her.

I invite you to look around and find a loving partner. A parent, wife, husband, brother, sister, boy or girlfriend. Find someone who loves you from the heart. If he/she really loves you, he/she will do anything for you. Life with diabetes will be much easier with a loving partner.

Exercise

Exercise, as we all know, has many benefits to our bodies, brains, heart, and soul. It is absolutely beneficial for people with diabetes as it helps them find a parallel passage to let go of some extra glucose. I tried weight training for a while but I found out that walking and swimming along with some push-ups and set-ups are the best sports suits my age and my condition. Both are gentle sports, and they feed my body and soul naturally.

A word of caution: I started brisk walking for one hour daily without fail. It has become my sacred hour. I call it the quality hour because it engages me calmly with the natural surrounding and releases stress so efficiently. Walking improves the condition of my respiratory, cardiovascular, and circulatory systems without putting too much pressure on my joints, unlike other heavier sports. Daily walking enhances my mental status after a long day of work and it reduces my insulin resistance for hours after doing it. I also swim once or twice weekly. The feeling you get after 30 minutes of swimming is incomparable with any other workout. One more thing that will add a value to your walking. Try to walk with your partner (husband/wife/friend, etc.). I walk with my wife, Rehab, every day. It allows us an environment of peaceful connection away from technology and other hassles at the end of the day.

It is worth mentioning that some people think 30 minutes or even one hour of exercise gives them the right to eat like monsters when they finish working out. Indeed, this is a huge mistake. Such practice hinders your weight control and it might negatively affect your blood sugar. This is especially true if you devour fast-acting carbs after exercise as it usually happens.

I would like to quote Dr. Jason Fung in his book Obesity Code about exercise, *"Diet and exercise have been prescribed as treatment for obesity as if they are equally important. But diet and exercise are not fifty-fifty partners like macaroni and cheese. Diet is Batman and exercise is Robin. Diet does 95 percent of the work and deserves all the attention; so logically, it would be sensible to focus on diet. Exercise is still healthy and important-just not equally important. It has many benefits, but weight loss is not among them. Exercise is like brushing your teeth. It is good for you and should be done every day. Just don't expect to lose weight."*[39]

So please finish your work out, drink water, take a shower, relax and eat healthy food with no starches or sugar. Enjoy your normal BS readings and you will realize you just discovered the happiness recipe.

Mental health

I do not allow diabetes to take me down. I face it bravely and work hard to keep my BS normal. I eat right and I exercise. And, I never hide that I am a diabetic. I always say, even though I am a diabetic but I am in 100% full control of it. Diabetes no longer intimidates me. Many PWD hide that they are diabetics, in work, neighborhood or in family! In my opinion, this is not right. There is nothing to shame the person with diabetes at all.

At work, I perform as everyone else does or even better. I remember I told my boss in my last job interview that I am an insulin-dependent diabetic but I am in total control of it and I perform better than any non-diabetic does. I didn't fear rejection or losing the job because I tell the truth and I have faith in myself.

I read voraciously and I am a prolific writer. This is my third book between your hands. I have no intention to stop writing and working. In fact, diabetes has improved my life. Yes, I admit the journey with diabetes is hard. It requires constant monitoring and real dedication. But, without a doubt, it has improved my eating habits, inspired me to start working out and gave me increased self-confidence knowing I can conquer such a monster.

Diabetes gave me the opportunity to reach out to PWD all over the world. It has granted me the courage to support and be there for whoever wants to learn about diabetes management. I always tell what I have learned and share my experience of controlling BS to the multitudes of people that need this information. Helping people makes one happy. Therefore, I do not resent diabetes, but I do not love it either. I realized I have to live with diabetes either in peace or in war. Therefore, I chose to live peacefully and not to allow diabetes to take away my physical or mental quality. Every time I opt for a good food choice and subsequently measure a normal blood sugar number, I consider that a great victory.

Chapter 12: Supplements

"Those of us with low HDL cholesterol are at far greater risk of having a heart attack than those of us with high total or LDL cholesterol."
Gary Taubes

I am not a fan of swallowing many supplements but I learned through research that some of them are of great significance for diabetics to take. I take Vitamin D, Magnesium, Vitamin C and Probiotics on a daily basis. I take B12, Chromium, Zinc, and Iodine periodically. I will talk about Magnesium, Vitamin D and Vitamin C here, which I think they help me in boosting my immune system and in reversing insulin resistance.

Magnesium

Most of the diabetics are deficient in Magnesium. Our bodies require 54 mg of magnesium to process 1 gram of sugar and starch.[40] In a study mentioned in the ADA site, Magnesium deficiency reduces insulin sensitivity and using Magnesium supplementation improves insulin sensitivity and metabolic control in subjects with T2 diabetes.[41] Magnesium is a cofactor in 300 enzymes systems in our bodies. Measuring Magnesium in the blood is not effective as 50 – 60% of it concentrated in bones, the rest in tissues and only 1% is circulating in the blood.

David Spero wrote in diabetes self-management website that according to Dr. Carolyn Dean, in her book <u>The Magnesium Miracle</u>, nearly 80% of Americans are deficient in Magnesium, and it is often the primary factor in heart disease, high blood pressure, diabetes, and most muscular problems.[4243]

I take 400 to 500 mg of Magnesium in the form of Magnesium glycinate or Citrate as our bodies absorb both efficiently. Many doctors recommend a higher dose than that. In her book Keto-Adapted, Maria Emmerich advised a daily dose of 400 – 1000 mg per day. She said, *"We mistakenly blame Cholesterol and saturated fats for heart disease, when it is really a magnesium deficiency. Studies have shown that adding 700 -1000 mg of magnesium glycinate helps decrease the rate of heart-associated death by 70%! I suggest at least 400 mg in the morning when blood pressure is the highest to help naturally relax constricted blood vessels"*[44] That shows how important Magnesium for heart health.

Magnesium is found in green leafy vegetables, avocados, raspberries, legumes, broccoli, cabbage, green beans, Brussels sprouts, salmon, and tuna fish.

Vitamin D

Many PWD suffer from vitamin D deficiency and I am one of them. In an epidemiological study published on April 19, 2018, conducted by California San Diego School of Medicine and Seoul National University suggests that individuals who are deficient in vitamin D may be at much greater risk in developing diabetes.[45]

"We found that participants with blood levels of 25-hydroxyvitamin D that were above 30 ng/ml had one-third of the risk of diabetes and those with levels above 50 ng/ml had one-fifth of the risk of developing diabetes," said first author Sue K. Park, MD, in the Department of Preventive Medicine at Seoul National University College of Medicine in South Korea.[46]

I take vitamin K2-MK7 along with vitamin D. Taking vitamin D alone doesn't allow the calcium to be absorbed in the right place. Instead of being absorbed in bones, it gets absorbed in tissues. Vitamin D along with vitamin K2 helps to correct this and directs the calcium absorption towards the right organ (bones). According to Dr. Alex Rinehart *"If you're looking for a baseline recommendation for D3 and K2 supplementation. 2000-5000IU of D3 ("cholecalciferol) and up to 320 mcg/day of vitamin K2-7 (found in Mega Quinone K2-7) are popular and safe ways to go as long as you're periodically checking at least your 25-OH vitamin D levels (storage; calcidiol)."*

Vitamin D boosts the immune system and reduces the risk of cancer. It also helps in reducing the episodes of getting colds and flu.

Dr. Cedric Garland of San Diego School of Medicine and Moores Cancer Center has published a paper saying that the risk of breast cancer could be cut by 50% if the serum level of vitamin D kept around 40 to 50 ng/ml.[47]

Vitamin D has a big role in disease prevention as it affects about 3000 genes out of the 30,000 genes in our bodies. Taking Vitamin D along with vitamin C, on a regular basis, greatly supports my immune system. Vitamin D level is controversy among doctors, while some doctors consider above 50 ng/ml is not safe, others see it completely safe. According to Maria Emmerich in Keto Adapted, below 50 ng/dl is too low despite the normal range of 30 ng/dl stated by most labs.[48]

I used to measure 15 ng/ml and accordingly, prescribed Vitamin D3 weekly injections for two months. This brings my vitamin D3 level to the normal range but unfortunately, the level gets down again after 6 months if I do not take a maintenance daily dose. So now, I keep a maintenance dose of 5000 IU daily all the time.

Vitamin C

Vitamin C boosts my immune system. I used to get flu every two months or so. Coincidently, I heard many videos to Dr. Andrew

Saul and others about the benefits of vitamin C to the immune system. I started taking it with high doses that reach to 10,000 to 15,000 mg when I feel the first symptoms of cold and it helps a lot for speedy recovery and reduction of colds and flu intensity. My normal daily dose of vitamin C is about 2000 to 3000 mg. Since taking vitamin C became a daily ritual, I don't get flu as much as before. And if it happens, it is never as severe.

Perhaps the story of side effects and kidney stones may pop up your mind while reading now. In order to clear this, I would like to quote Dr. Andrew Saul here *"Vitamin C is remarkably safe even in enormously high doses. Compared to commonly used prescription drugs, side effects are virtually nonexistent. It does not cause kidney stones. In fact, vitamin C increases urine flow and favorably lowers the pH to help keep stones from forming. William J. McCormick, M.D. used vitamin C since the late 1940's to prevent and treat kidney stones. Vitamin C does not significantly raise oxalate levels, and uric acid stones have never resulted from its use, either. Said Dr. Klenner: "The ascorbic acid/kidney stone story is a myth."*[49]

If you like to know more about vitamin C, please listen to Dr. Andrew's videos on YouTube.

Chapter 13: Robert who saved me

"So for breakfast, you could have a bowl of cornflakes with no added sugar, or a bowl of sugar with no added cornflakes. They would taste different but, below the neck, act more or less the same."
Dr. David Ludwig

My seat came next to him on my flight heading to Stuttgart, Germany to attend a business seminar. He was a German man, as I learned later, in his mid-forties half-bald with small circular glasses, which adds a tinge of virtual intelligence to his face. He looked disheveled, erratic, and fidgeting in an impatient and restless manner. I did not pay much attention to him. I was thinking deeply about the intruder who showed up aggressively into my life lately. What will I do with this silent killer that attacked me suddenly? Diabetes has introduced me to nearly a dozen doctors and a plethora of new medications.

Basically, I was given ordinary mainstream medical advice. I discovered later that most of this advice did not help me to achieve normal blood sugar. I also figured out later that the dilapidated guidelines, I was preached about, caused fatal complications and severe suffering for many people with diabetes all over the world.

Unfortunately, I could not control my diabetes at all, despite all the efforts I had put in to carefully follow their instructions.

In general, I am an obedient patient. Nevertheless, my blood sugar numbers were always high and uncontrollable. I committed to reading about diabetes management. I looked around at bookstores to find a good book about diabetes management in Arabic, but I found nothing of value. Most of the books were interpretations of the ADA guidelines.

Suddenly, I was brought back from my pondering about diabetes by the sound of the flight host asking me: "Would you like something to drink, sir?"

I answered: "Yes, natural orange juice without sugar please," and then went on smugly completing the sentence "because I am diabetic!"

The guy next to me flounced angrily, looked at me censurably and asked: "What did you just say? Are you diabetic and drinking juice?"

I said, "Yes, I drink a natural healthy juice without any added sugar."

He said, "Even if it is natural and without sugar! Don't you know that one glass of orange juice contains least 4 to 5 squeezed oranges and each orange has about 20 grams of carbohydrates (between glucose and fructose)? The glucose part will raise your blood sugar about 50 to 60 mg/dl per one orange as per your weight? Now, when you squeeze all these oranges you only get the sugar and strip out all the fibers that come naturally with the orange to delay the absorption of sugar in it! You will just drink the sugar in five oranges by doing this. What could possibly be natural about this! I am not even talking about the negative effect of the huge amount of fructose you are about to sip! Without a doubt, drinking such juice will raise your blood sugar massively and rapidly. You know what? I will do you a favor you will never forget."

"Why is this person so interested in helping me? Something seems weird here! And, what are these algorithms he is talking about! Carbohydrates, sugar, glucose, fructose, fiber? This seems deranged. Let me see where this conversation will lead." Talking to myself!

With an unmistakable look of defiance, he reached into his bag and took a big book out of it. He paused a little and said politely, "Please take this book and just read it until our plane lands in Stuttgart and I will take it back from you before we say goodbye." Then he handed me a big book of 511 pages. His eyes were talking to me silently as if he wanted to say, "Please do yourself a favor and read this book before diabetes kills you."

"Is this man for real? Is he really thinking I could read such a big book before we land?" Talking to myself again.

To my amazement, it seemed he just read my mind and knew what I was thinking, as he suddenly said, "Believe me, you really need to read this book. It will improve your life and many other lives. So, please start immediately and do not waste time."

The book title was "Dr. Bernstein's Diabetes Solution" by Dr. Richard K. Bernstein. I wondered who is this Dr. Richard Bernstein?

One hour had already passed from the long eight hours flight. I put on my headphones to listen to some music played by my favorite pianist, Omar Khairat. For a moment, I was curious to know about the author's solution for diabetes. Simultaneously, I felt no desire to read about diabetes now. It has been really tedious squeezing diabetes into every corner of my life. Besides, I knew there was no use in reading such books, as diabetes is a progressive disease anyway and no matter what I do, I will inevitably deteriorate. That was the repeated warning I always hear from my doctor.

Therefore, I pretended I am reading until my new friend falls asleep, so I can go to sleep as well. I opened the book to a random page and it so happened that this page was about complications of uncontrolled diabetes, specifically, the diabetic foot. I felt more anxious and averse and I wanted to put the book aside and sleep. I began to hear the sound of little snoring. Finally, my friend had taken a comfortable decision, for both of us. He took off his shoes, crossed his legs in a relaxed way and slept.

Relieved, I thought, Thank God." Let us wait another five minutes until he starts dreaming. Then I will place the book aside and sleep like a baby. While getting ready to execute my plan, my eyes fall on something strange. Part of my friend's upper foot that was placed over the other seemed very hard and full. It seemed artificial.

I rubbed my eyes and then looked at his foot again. But, yeah, it was abnormal. Something was wrong. My heart was pounding rapidly with a background of escalating snoring from beside me. All of the sudden, I decided to touch his foot lightly to see if my eyes were right or wrong. I acted as if I was going to the restroom. I stood up and touched his feet gently as I passed by while on my way out to the corridor. OMG! Yes, I was right! It was wood, steel or anything, but it was not a normal foot.

Oh, the guy's foot was amputated. Could it be one of the diabetes complications resulted from poor control of his diabetes? That must be why he insisted I read and learn, so I can avoid such a fate!

I turned back to my seat and mesmerized for a moment. I was riveted there for five long minutes. While I was sweating and thinking, the man opened his eyes, as if he knew exactly what happened. He disclosed a sad smile while saying, through misty eyes, "learn before turning back becomes impossible".

With silent involuntary overflowing tears, I opened the book from the beginning and started to read. And, from the first page, I knew this book was different. Just 15 minutes of reading and I became an addict. Oh My God, what is this? Clear, smooth, convincing and profuse science? Dr. Richard Bernstein is an Eighty-three years old physician and a genius Engineer who was diagnosed with T1 diabetes at the age of 12. He was on the verge of death at the age of forty suffering from all possible complications, despite following what doctors advised him (The ADA guidelines).

He discovered the secret of controlling his diabetes by cutting all fast-acting carbohydrates. His daily consumption of carbs never exceeded 30 grams of slow-acting carbohydrate. He added a basal insulin strategy to his treatment. Finally, he got his diabetes under control and started reaping the benefits of normal BS. Most of his painful complications reversed. He tried to spread the word to help people with diabetes all over the world but, in fact, he found himself fighting against the medical establishment. He was swimming against the strong current of low fat/high carb diet media and industry.

He expected to be attacked and silenced because he was not a physician. So, he decided to become a doctor. He went to medical school at the age of forty-five and graduated as a physician at the age of fifty. Of course, he reversed most of his complications by normalizing his blood sugar. He became one of the best physicians who achieve unprecedented results with his patients. Fortunately, he wrote this magnificent book in my hand that, literally, would change my whole life.

I was consumed by this great book until I felt Robert's hand patting on my shoulder while saying, "Only 15 minutes to land my friend." OMG, I had spent nearly seven hours reading without realizing the time. I had finished two-thirds of the book. This book had planted the seeds of magic in me. It had already changed my life for the better. It completely altered my attitude in dealing with diabetes forever: it gave me *hope*

We landed and I hugged my friend Robert who had saved me indeed. The goodbye was full of tears out of gratefulness to this great person.

Robert dedicated the book to me and wrote down some words that always provoke my tears any time I read them. He wrote, *"From a friend with one foot to a friend with two feet, please keep your feet attached."*

My friend Robert guided me to the right track and gave me a real example of how to help people out of love and kindness. Thank you dear Robert - You have saved my life and the lives of many.

Chapter 14: Are you Diabetic and don't know it

"Doctors put drugs of which they know little into bodies of which they know less for diseases of which they know nothing at all."
Voltaire

For every two people with diabetes, one of them is still undiagnosed. There are 316 million people in the world have glucose intolerance and are on their way to getting diabetes if they do not take an action to reverse it. So, is it possible you are diabetic or pre-diabetic and you have no clue about it? The diagnosis of T2 diabetes often happens after experiencing some obvious symptoms such as frequent urination, extreme thirst, losing weight. If you experienced one or all of these symptoms, you definitely waited too long and most possibly, you are diabetic by now. In fact, I was diagnosed with a blood sugar of 420 mg/dl after having all these symptoms, which escalated gradually, for almost an entire year.

In one of Dr. Bernstein's university YouTube videos, he mentioned that many newly diagnosed T2 patients, who came to his clinic for the first time, already had several diabetes complications. This means they suffered from slightly elevated blood sugar for a year or two before been diagnosed. That is why it is crucial to watch out for the very early symptoms before you reach the revealing ones. If your weight creeps up, if you crave sugar and starches or if you stop moving and exercising, then you need to worry. You must take whatever measures needed to reverse this condition before it worsens.

You can guess your odds of having insulin resistance / metabolic syndrome (and later T2 diabetes) if you have one or more of the following symptoms.

- Extreme hunger.
- Excessive desire for starches, sweets, juices, Sodas, etc.
- Midsection (belly) fat.
- Slightly elevated blood pressure.
- Slightly elevated fasting blood sugar.
- High Triglyceride levels.
- Glucose intolerance one or two hours after eating starches or sugary food.
- Elevated fasting blood sugar.
- If one of your parents or a close relative has T2 diabetes.

These are all symptoms of metabolic syndrome (MS) which, most likely, if not reversed, will turn to full-blown T2 diabetes. If you have one or more of these symptoms, you need to act immediately. Acting early after the discovery of metabolic syndrome (MS) symptoms could delay or even reverse the inevitable diagnosis of T2 diabetes. In many occasions, one can be able to reverse MS completely with some basic changes in food intake and activity level or even by intermittent fasting. Unfortunately, MS early symptoms are usually left undetected.

Assume you noticed some of those symptoms early enough and decided to act on them before they act on you. You consulted a mainstream physician immediately who gives you the conventional advice "exercise, minimize fat intake, add the so-called healthy grains, and fruits"

Next, your physician will compare your blood sugar numbers to American Diabetes Association guidelines' numbers and he will consider them perfect or at least within the acceptable range. He/she will definitely tell you the famous sentence "you are on the borderline." Ironically, the BS numbers they consider acceptable are not, simply because they are not normal BS numbers. Those numbers will admit you into the type 2 diabetes club in no time. Therefore, you need to be aware that mainstream "borderline" level are T2 diabetes level already. Do not wait for this to happen and act immediately.

Let me give you an example: Assume your Fasting BS is 122 mg/dl. According to the ADA, the pre-diabetes fasting BS range is up to 126 mg/dl. Your physician will warn you that you are on the borderline and you must watch your food intake (eat right) and start to exercise. Actually, the real normal Fasting BS is between 75 to 90 mg/dl. A study mentioned in Jenny Ruhl's book <u>Blood Sugar 101</u> stated that people who measured fasting BS of 92 mg/dl or above are much more likely to develop T2 diabetes within a decade.[50] Even though your physician may tell you, normal fasting blood sugar is 100 mg/dl and the borderline is 126 mg/dl. Therefore, if you read a fasting blood sugar of 92 mg/dl or above, act immediately to fix this.

Obviously, you do not want to wait until you become glucose intolerant or reach a fasting blood sugar of 110 or 120 to act. Do not listen to any mainstream physician in this regard. You instantly need to cut fast-acting carbohydrates, reduce weight, increase your activity level and consult a physician who believes in the importance of keeping normal blood sugar levels. If you do so, you probably will reverse the metabolic syndrome and avoid getting T2 diabetes. When it comes to diabetes management, never buy the "take it easy attitude", never.

I would also advise you to do the fasting insulin level lab test. It will reveal whether you have insulin resistance. The person with insulin resistance secretes much more insulin compared to a normal person. Fasting insulin level test can provide early information on whether you are prone to develop metabolic syndrome.

According to the International Diabetes Federation (IDF), poor control of diabetes killed 4.9 million in 2014 alone. There is a diabetic person dies every seven seconds because of poor control of diabetes. Spending on diabetes treatment reached 727 Billion US Dollars in 2017 as compared to 673 in 2016.[51] These are scary numbers and a real economic burden. They actually represent a loss of money, health, and productivity.

Despite that, 77% of People with diabetes are from poor countries but the spending on treatment is always higher in modern and western countries, which have 23% of the global count of People with diabetes. NAC (North America and The Caribbean's) annual expenditure on diabetes is 377 Billion US dollars, which, alone, represents 52% on the world expenditure on diabetes.

So start your prevention plan now, especially if you live in one of those unfortunate countries that spend little on diabetes treatment. Take the decision of skipping every food raises your blood sugar and let your meter judge your choices. Redefine whether the food is healthy by its direct effect on your blood sugar. You do this and you will save yourself a big headache.

Chapter 15: T1 diabetes kids

"What if I, a physician, told you, a diabetic, to eat a diet that consisted of 60 percent sugar, 20 percent protein and 20 percent fat? More than likely, you'd think I was insane. I'd think I was insane, and I would never make this suggestion to a diabetic (nor would I even make it to a nondiabetic)."
Dr. Richard K. Bernstein

The most distressing thing about kids with T1 diabetes is how lightly the management of their diabetes taken by many parents and physicians. Management of anything should be result oriented. So, if the T1 diabetes management plan brings uncontrolled blood sugar numbers, then other plans have to be considered until achieving tight BS control. Since T1 kids are diagnosed with diabetes at a younger age, it is expected they will live a longer duration having T1 diabetes. This duration will be so painful and hard without excellent control. If we assume someone will live to the age of 75 and that he was diagnosed with diabetes at age 35, so he will live 40 years with diabetes. While a T1 kid, who was diagnosed at the age of two is expected to live 73 years with diabetes if we assume he will live up to 75. If the control is not stringent, the consequences will be terrible, considering the long duration.

Many kids with T1 diabetes are not even close to achieving normal blood sugar. There are many practices, and sometimes myths, encourage keeping T1 kids in the abnormal blood sugar range. Most times, the concept of normal blood sugar is not even considered in the minds of the circle around the T1 kid, whether they are parents, physicians, diabetes educators or nutritionists. I usually get messages from mothers of T1 kids had been told that normal blood sugar of non-diabetic kids (supposed to be the target for T1 kid) runs higher than adults' normal BS! On the contrary, Dr. Bernstein said that normal BS for kids actually runs a bit lower than normal BS of adults. Let me shed some light on some facts and misconceptions about the management of T1 kids with diabetes.

Kids are very sensitive to insulin

A three-year-old kid may have a correction factor of 150 to 200 (i.e. each fast-acting insulin unit may lower his/her BS about 150 to 200 mg/dl). In his book, Think like a Pancreas Gary Scheiner mentioned that the correction factor value for someone with total daily insulin of seven units would be between 220 – 260. This will be almost any 1 to 2-year-old T1 kid. So, if we assume that the sleeping time blood sugar for this kid is 200 mg/dl and the normal blood sugar we need to bring him down to, is between 80 to 100 mg/dl, such mission will be impossible using one unit of FAI otherwise his blood sugar will drop to zero.

An insulin pump user could use decimals of insulin unit and correct his/her BS, in this case. However, this solution is only available for T1 kids in rich countries where medical insurance covers the pump cost. Sadly, in many parts of the world, an insulin pump does not even exist in the diabetes management dictionary. It is a dream impossible to be achieved. Other solutions, to bring his/her BS down, are insulin dilution or by using the half-unit pen that could enable half-unit injection. However, even the half-unit is still considered a high dose for many cases where more correction precisely needed (for example from 140 mg/dl to 90 mg/dl with a correction factor of 200). Assuredly, many physicians know nothing about insulin dilution and some consider it an outdated method!

On the other hand, physicians usually rationalize keeping the blood sugar of the T1 kid high. They are scared from the hypoglycemia episodes that might happen to high-insulin-sensitive-T1 kids due to BS correction. Unfortunately, the majority of physicians advise the mothers of T1 kids to let him/her sleep at 200 mg/dl to avoid hypoglycemia. Accordingly, many kids with T1 diabetes are left with high blood sugar most of the time, which is devastating indeed. Fast forward, when complications strike, the physician will come up with their famous sentence, "It is a progressive disease!"

T1 kids also are very sensitive to carbohydrates

T1 kids can't process carbohydrates without the use of external insulin but the manufactured insulin is never the same efficiency as natural pancreas insulin. T1 kids are very sensitive to carbohydrates, especially the fast-acting carbohydrates. One gram of carbohydrates raises my BS about 4 mg/dl. So, if I eat 30 grams of carbs, it would raise my blood sugar about 120 mg/dl. While the same one gram of FAC raises a 3-year-old kid, about 15 mg/dl and the 30 grams of FAC will raise his BS about 450 mg/dl! In brief, the negative effect of the high carb diet on blood sugar of T1 kid is very clear because of their high sensitivity to carbs and to insulin.

Because of such sensitivity to both carbohydrates and insulin, a T1 kid's blood sugar, who eats a high starchy diet, is always severely fluctuating up and down. Any small mistake could lead to an unstable or dangerously low BS.

- Mistakes in carbs' count.
- Wrong insulin timing.
- Wrong IC ratio.
- Wrong consideration of IOB, if any.

- The speed of insulin absorption in related to various body injection spots.
- Any unexpected delay in digestion.
- Any food label error.
- Hypoglycemia may happen if the child exercises right after a meal without considering a reduction in meal insulin.

All these factors are magnified when the carbohydrates intake per meal is high. The combination of high carb foods, high insulin and high probabilities of errors is a real recipe for a tough life for the T1 diabetes kid. It is so important to break such a vicious circle by eating the food that doesn't raise BS in the first place or at least raises it gradually not sharply.

As a parent of T1 kid, you will always listen to things as carbs is so important for his/her growth, you cannot cut carbs, etc. I stopped arguing about this topic as I believe the desire to achieve tight diabetes control is a choice to be taken by the family of T1 child. Some families insist on strict control and some other families are ok with mediocre control. At the end, every choice has consequences. However, I would only mention a couple of things I am 100% sure about, in my opinion:

1. There will be no benefit from any food raises blood sugar, as the harms of high blood sugar outweigh any expected benefit from such food. This is a governing rule I always use it to control my blood sugar. What is the benefit of eating a piece of bread that raises my blood sugar to 300s even for only 15 minutes! Damage is done.
2. The glucometer should be the judge whether the food, any diabetic eats, is good for his/her blood sugar or no. **My sincere advice to parents of T1 child: don't listen to no one, not even Dr. Bernstein or whoever, just let your meter talks and take the decision accordingly**. It is that simple.
3. Who said T1 Kids would stop eating all carbs? They will only need to avoid the fast-acting carbohydrates and they will definitely eat slow-acting carbs like leafy vegetables

and berries for example. So, even if someone argues about the necessity of carbs, the answer is: he/she will definitely eats carbs, but only the one that gradually raises his/her blood sugar (not sharply) because he/she can't tolerate the fast acting ones.

4. The ultimate goal for any parents of T1 kid is to grow him/her up as healthy, young man/woman free of any complications. You and I know that this will only happen if he/she keeps a normal BS all the time. If you heartily realize this, you will do whatever it takes to achieve that goal. Just believe in this goal and act accordingly.

It is not that I have a tunnel vision when it comes to low carb WOE, not at all. I never had the tendency to exclude any other option if it works and bring great results. I am just saying T1 kid (or any diabetic indeed) needs to eat under the umbrella of an ultimate goal of achieving normal blood sugar all the time, so he can avoid developing complications later on. Logically, which is better? Living the whole day with BS between 80 to 120 mg/dl or between 50 to 400 mg/dl! Considering my personal experience, the low carb WOE is the only way enables me, and many PWD I know, to precisely control our blood sugar. I tried every other way, but it did not work with me at all. Well if you slack a bit in eating carbohydrates, your BS control will slack as well. In the end, we are human and it is not a fight; who is right and who is wrong. It is a choice.

Hypoglycemia and T1 kids?

As I said, T1 kids are too sensitive to insulin. With such high insulin sensitivity, a mistake of injecting one extra unit of insulin is fatal. This is why injecting much of it will cause high odds of getting hypoglycemia. Dr. Bernstein called it industrial doses of insulin. Therefore, T1 kid, who eats a high carb diet, will inject a relatively high amount of insulin, which will rapidly cause the vicious circle of lows and highs during the twenty-four hours. This is something commonly seen in many kids with T1 diabetes. As per the low of small numbers of Dr. Bernstein, "the less carb T1 eats, the less insulin he/she injects, the smaller the mistakes could happen and the easier to be fixed."

Following the plan of Dr. Bernstein of 30 grams/day of slow-acting carbohydrates and adequate protein along with natural fat that comes with it, will not only normalize blood sugar but it will also stabilize it with rare incidents of hypoglycemia and hyperglycemia. I remember how my life was miserable while eating a high carb diet. My normal daily pattern was a continuous episode of high and low blood sugar.

The Typeonegrit study

Many doctors still warn their diabetic patients to avoid healthy fat and push them to consume the standard high carbohydrates diet, whole grains, Complex carbohydrates, starchy food, and fruits. They just do not let go the same old practice even it brings miserable BS results. They still turn their eyes blind on the good control results from following the low carb, adequate protein, and healthy fat WOE compared to high carb, low fat one.

I would like here to refer to a very promising study published on May 7th, 2018,[52] led by Belinda Lennerz, MD, Ph.D., and David Ludwig, MD, Ph.D., of Boston Children's Hospital. Participants Patients were mostly T1 diabetics and were drawn from typeonegrit Facebook group. Typeonegrit is a Facebook group with about 3000 members and following the recommendations of Dr. Richard Bernstein explained in details in his book Dr. Bernstein's diabetes solution. The group is an advocate for a low carb diet approach to manage T1 diabetes. Two-third of members have an HbA1c less than 5.9%. 316 participants provided enough information out of 493 subjects took the survey. Forty-two percent of the participants were children with T1 diabetes.

Participants reported average daily carbohydrates consumption of 36 grams, which represents around 5% of their total daily calories. Of course, you can see the difference between this and the 45% of daily calories of carbs recommended by ADA.

The finding was amazing. The study found that the HbA1c average fell down from 7.15% to an amazing 5.67% with a very few hospitalizations of hypoglycemia. Such results cannot be obtained with a high carb diet. Tight control requires less carbohydrate intake and continuous monitoring of blood sugar, which almost all group members were committed to. I am a proud member of this informative group and one of the founders of this group, Rd Dikeman,[53] had written me the foreword of my first book What You Don't Know about Diabetes (written in Arabic). I would like to grasp the chance to thank the admins of this magnificent group for the great efforts they do in supporting PWD all over the world. Thank you, Allison Herschede, Rd Dikeman, Derek C. Raulerson and Debbie Wright Theriault. I also participated in this study with my results and daily routine.

Positive change in the ADA attitude

On December 17th, 2018 the American Diabetes Association released its new 2019 Lifestyle Standard of Medical Care in Diabetes.[54] ADA continued to change its approach towards diabetes management. Now ADA states the following on their website, *"In addition, research indicates that Low carbohydrate eating plans may result in improving glycemia and have the potential to reduce antihyperglycemic medications for type two diabetes."* I believe they will include T1 in the near future because it is the same concept.

ADA also mentioned, *"Evidence suggests that there is not an ideal percentage of calories from carbohydrate, protein, and fat for all people with diabetes. Therefore, macronutrient distribution should be based on an individualized assessment of current eating patterns, preferences, and metabolic goals. Consider personal preferences (e.g., tradition, culture, religion, health beliefs and goals, economics) as well as metabolic goals when working with individuals to determine the best eating pattern for them."* ADA also mentioned, *"As research studies on some low-*

carbohydrate eating plans generally indicate challenges with long-term sustainability, it is important to reassess and individualize meal plan guidance regularly for those interested in this approach."

Of course, I disagree with this here as the rate of adherence to low carb is high and I am (and many others) an example of this. Following it for the past 8 years and going. However, such a positive change in the ADA approach is encouraging and promising with better diabetes management approaches in the near future.

Until then, our T1 kids with diabetes are a treasure that we have to keep and nurture. We need to keep them always in normal blood sugar range so they can live healthy lives.

Chapter 16: Omar and Sara

"What mostly raises blood sugar—and for most of us this is the only thing that raises blood sugar—is eating starch and sugar. Cut back on them, and your blood sugar will plummet immediately."
Jenny Ruhl

With her beautiful eyes and charming smile, Sara captured Omar's heart the first time he saw her in college. She, pretty much, looks like his sister Doaa in her vigor, soft seriousness, and politeness. Every time he lays an eye on her with a pounding heart, her face shines with a soft smile and she then turns the other side out of shyness. Sara is an orphan. She lives alone with her mother after her father passed away when she was four years old. She has no siblings. Her single mother works hard to support the small family.

The situation wasn't any different for Sara. She also has her heart filled with this handsome young man. Every time she passes by, she feels his gazes at her. She sees him as a loving kind giant. With his respectful and loving character, her heart was taken already.

Omar was so keen not to disclose his love now until he graduates. Involuntarily, his eyes always tell his inside. It was kind of Platonic love indeed. He just kept a promise to himself that if he will ever get married, then his wife will be Sara and no one else.

Days passed, Omar graduated and became a junior engineer. He opened the issue with his parents and asked them to bless his request to be engaged with Sara. After getting their approval, he arranged a family visit to Sara's house on Wednesday night. Sara's heart was dancing after hearing the news about the expected visit. She called Omar the night before the visit and told him, "Omar, there is something I want to talk to you about; something about me you should know now before you show up here with your family tomorrow. Something might let you change your mind."

"No, I do not want to know anything, I already know enough to choose you to be my wife forever, I will see you tomorrow Sara, bye now," Omar said.

On Wednesday, Omar, his sister Doaa, and his parents showed up on time for the eagerly anticipated visit. Sara's mother welcomed them with a big smile and started talking chummy and friendly. Then suddenly Sara interrupted the conversation and looked at Omar and his family saying, "there is something important you all should know before we talk about engagement arrangement. Something even Omar did not know, I tried to tell him but he refused to listen." Everyone was all ears waiting what Sara has to say.

"I am a type one diabetic," Sara said starting with a little sigh. And immediately she added with a confident voice, "but I am in complete control of my diabetes." It seemed Omar did not care, as he loved Sara with or without diabetes. However, parent's faces got colored instantly. For a moment, the environment was fraught with silence. A few minutes later, Omar's family excused themselves to leave with a trivial promise that they will be back later to discuss the engagement details! Sadly, they never show up again.

Sara spent the whole night and the following nights crying. Sleep flew out of her eyes forever. What happened broke her heart and crushed her soul. On the other side, Omar wasn't in better condition than her. All his efforts to get his parents to approve the marriage failed. With a narrow mind mentality and ignorant attitude, his parents thought, "why should our son ties his life with someone with a serious illness like T1 diabetes?"

Two years passed by, so slowly, and Sara is in her last year at college already. Walking around with eyes no more bright and heart filled with sadness and pain. Until one fine day, Sara's home bell rang. She opened up the door to be met with a big surprise! Omar's parents and Doaa came to visit. "OMG, what brought them again after all that happened," Sara talked to herself.

She couldn't do better than cold welcoming. She called her mother to come over and join them. One silent minute passed, and no one is talking until Omar's father broke down in tears and said regrettably, "Sara please forgive us. Omar's mother and I committed a huge mistake and we are here to fix it. In short, One week ago, we accidently discovered that my daughter Doaa had type one diabetes. We realized that having T1 diabetes is something out of any one hand. Unfortunately, we learned the hard way. And here we are, between your hands to apologize to you for our selflessness and our narrow minds. I want you to realize that there is no one on the face of earth loves you more than Omar, he really does. Since that day, Omar was always in ongoing dissension with us and it turned out he was right and we were wrong."

Sara was sitting there speechless and holding herself not to cry. Suddenly, the bell rang again, and it was Omar. When she saw Omar, Sara's heart almost leaped out of her chest and finally, her smile shone up again behind her misty eyes. She stood up, caught Doaa hand, and said loudly, "Come with me to my room Doaa and let me teach you how to control your T1 diabetes."

Chapter 17: Insulin makes you fat

"The higher the blood glucose after consumption of food, the greater the insulin level, the more fat is deposited. This is why, say, eating a three-egg omelet that triggers no increase in glucose does not add to body fat, while two slices of whole wheat bread increases blood glucose to high levels, triggering insulin and growth of fat, particularly abdominal or deep visceral fat."
Dr. William Davis.

I nsulin makes you fat. Insulin has a direct relationship with the fat around your belly and everywhere else in your body. Insulin is a fat hormone, as it is not only concerned about clearing glucose from the bloodstream, as most of us know, but it is also concerned about fat storage and release.

Dr. Jason Fung said in his book <u>Obesity Code</u>, *"Actually, I can make anybody fat. How? By prescribing insulin. It won't matter that you have willpower, or that you exercise. It's simply a matter of enough insulin and enough time."*[55] In fact, when it comes to fat accumulation, insulin is the maestro. It is the main regulator of metabolism in our bodies. To understand the relationship between insulin and fat, we need to discuss some enzymes that are always influenced by the existence of insulin in the bloodstream.

Lipoprotein Lipase (LPL)

LPL is the main answer to the repeated question of why do men and women get fat in different areas of the body? Men get fat stored around the waist and less on other areas while women get fat accumulated in the rear, thighs, and less on other areas in most cases.

LPL is an enzyme exists on the outer surface of muscles and fatty (adipose) tissues. It allows fatty acids and glucose to enter the fat cells and combine inside to form Triglyceride (the storage form of fat in our bodies). If the LPL on the fat cells is more active than the LPL on the muscles cells, then the body will tend to accumulate more fat than burning it as a fuel in muscles cells. In short, people with a high response of adipose tissue's LPL to high carb diet, and accordingly high insulin, will gain fat easily.[56]

Insulin, the motivator

Insulin is the major motivator of LPL activity. This is considered one function of insulin in the direction of metabolism regulation. The existence of insulin in the bloodstream activates LPL on adipose tissue. Accordingly, more fat will be stored on our fat cells. When blood sugar goes up, the pancreas releases insulin stored in its granules or secretes more of it, if needed, to deal immediately with the rise of glucose. In fact, this is the first priority of insulin. Insulin will do anything to perform this mission perfectly and keep the extra glucose (energy) away from the bloodstream. In the meantime, any other source of energy, rather than glucose, has to be relegated for some time until the case with extra glucose is resolved. This is well understood because high blood glucose is toxic to our organs.

Part of the glucose in our bloodstream is used to supply energy to cells as needed. Part of the rest replenishes the glycogen stores in muscles and liver as a stand by energy used when required. The rest is pushed into fat cells via insulin signal to LPL and get converted to glycerol, which combines with three molecules of fatty acids forming Triglyceride.

If we minimize the carbohydrate intake, the insulin will be decreased in our bloodstream and the LPL will be deactivated. This allows TG to be decomposed and liberated to its main components and then carried by lipoproteins through the bloodstream to various parts of our bodies for usage. This also happens with the aid of an enzyme called sensitive Lipase (HSL).

Hormone-Sensitive Lipase (HSL)

Insulin also influences another enzyme (HSL) that has a big role in helping our bodies burn more of our stored fat. HSL makes fat cells less fatty by breaking down TG into its main components of fatty acids and glucose and releases them to the bloodstream.

Conclusively, if insulin is present in our bloodstream, it activates LPL to store more fat and deactivates HSL to prevent liberating stored fat. All that for the sake of the two pieces of double-glazed donut you devoured that raised your blood sugar, Insulin levels, and the stored fat as well!

Logically, if carbohydrate provokes insulin secretion, which launches the process of fat storage, does this means T1 diabetics need to give up injecting insulin? Absolutely no, insulin is mandatory in all T1 cases. The key is to minimize the fast-acting carbohydrates intake, so T1 person can minimize the total number of insulin units injected. Accordingly, avoid the vicious circle mentioned above as much as possible.

To understand this better, let me elaborate a bit about the types of insulin people with T1 diabetes inject. Basically, there are two groups of insulin:

Fast/Short-acting insulin (FAI) or bolus insulin

Fast-acting insulin, Novolog (Novorapid), Apidra or Humalog or short-acting insulin (regular insulin) like Humulin R. or Actrapid here in the Middle East. Fast-acting insulin peaks in about 30 – 60 minutes and ends from the bloodstream in about 3 to 4 hours. This varies from one to another. While short-acting insulin peaks slower in about 90 to 150 minutes and it ends from the bloodstream in about 5 hours, which is apparently slower than FAI.

Fast or short-acting insulin are injected before, with or after food according to the type of meal. The higher the glycemic index and load of the food, the more time needed for injection prior to eating. Please note that you can inject FAI at the same time or even after eating very low glycemic food. With protein, for example, I inject FAI (Novorapid) 20 to 30 minutes after eating. With leafy vegetables, I inject it while eating. Rarely, when my meal has rice, pasta, bread or potatoes, I inject FAI 15 to 20 minutes before eating. Dr. Bernstein prefers using the regular insulin and it works fine with many people adopting low carb WOE because it matches the gradual rise in BS resulted from such food. Anyway, I prefer using the FAI and play with injection timing.

Long / intermediate-acting insulin or basal insulin

Long-acting basal insulin such as Lantos, Tresiba, Levemir or intermediate insulin (NPH insulin) like Humulin N or Insultard in the Middle East. Basal insulin (also called background insulin) is injected once, twice and sometimes thrice every twenty-four hours. Basal insulin should stabilize your blood sugar while fasting, during sleep time or between meals. It gives a periodical tiny amount of insulin to cover the glucose released by the liver. In this way, energy could reach our cells and our organs can find the fuel to operate.

Quantity and frequency of basal units vary from one to another according to basal real-life needs. Dr. Bernstein, for example, advises to divide Levemir to three doses every twenty-four hours as follows: once in the morning, once at 10 pm and once at two am. In addition, he advises dividing Tresiba to two doses per 24 hours. Again, this varies between you and me, as we are different. While once every 24 hours of Tresiba works well with me, I know many T1 divide Tresiba to two doses every 24 hours and this works perfectly with them as well.

Intermediate insulin lasts about 10 hours or less and it has a moderate peak that can cause hypoglycemia if not carefully monitored. About six years ago, I used intermediate insulin for about three months, but it did not work well for me. Now a day, when I am off the insulin pump, I am doing great using Tresiba once every 24 hours with four or five units of NPH at 11 pm to conquer the dawn phenomenon. When I am fasting, the Tresiba does the trick alone because of diminished glycogen storage.

How you lose weight while injecting insulin

This is not an easy mission because the more insulin you inject the fatter you will be especially if you are an insulin-dependent T2. Many people with T2 diabetes are more prone to gain weight and have difficulty losing it with the use of insulin. It is the same for those with LADA as they are insulin resistant as well but in a lesser form than T2 fellows are. On the other hand, many people with T1 diabetes are more sensitive to insulin, so they don't gain weight easily with the use of insulin.

T2 comes from a background of insulin resistance (IR) for years. Therefore, they usually use more insulin to control their blood sugar to overcome the IR. I know many insulin-dependent T2 who always wonder how such tiny amount of insulin can control their T1 fellows' blood sugar compared to them. The answer is, T1 people are more sensitive to insulin.

Unquestionably, the key to losing weight while using insulin is to minimize insulin usage or secretion as much as possible by eating low carb food and intermittent fasting. Just bear in mind that this task should never be at the expense of messing up your blood sugar. I cannot emphasize enough that keeping normal blood sugar is of primary importance to living a good life as a person with diabetes.

The only way to reduce insulin is to reduce the food that makes you inject or secrete more insulin if you are T1 or T2, respectively. However, this will only occur when you cut all fast-acting carbohydrates. Committed to this alone, enabled me to reduce my daily bolus about 70% and it made a large positive difference in my ability to normalize my BS together with keeping my weight always in check. **While eating high carb food, I used to inject at least 60 units per twenty-four hours of Novorapid compared to 15 units only when adopted low carb WOE.**

If you combine low carb WOE along with 24 hours intermittent fasting at least twice a week, it will support you in reducing both fast-acting and basal insulin. Intermittent fasting depletes most of the glycogen stores, which assists in not only reducing bolus insulin but also reducing basal insulin as well. Based on my own experience, intermittent fasting made it possible for me to reduce basal insulin around 30%, as long as I keep fasting at least thrice a week twenty-four hours each.

Furthermore, if you add exercise to intermittent fasting and low carbs WOE, your insulin sensitivity will dramatically improve. Add some moderate weight training along with 60 minutes daily walk, alternative days, about five to six days a week and you will see great results. Of course, you need to consult your physician in case if you have any kidney, eye or foot complications before starting any exercise program. I walk 60 mins a day for 6 days a week and it is very beneficial, along with good food choices, for my blood sugar, insulin sensitivity, and overall wellbeing.

Before the discovery of insulin, diabetes was named the melting disease. At that time, T1 diabetes diagnosis was like a death sentence. So, insulin is a gift to people with diabetes. You just need to deal with it very sensibly because too much of it harms our bodies, same as glucose. Exactly.

Chapter 18: Losing weight for insulin-dependents

"The simple answer as to why we get fat is that carbohydrates make us so; protein and fat do not"

Gary Taubes

Dr. Robert H. Lustig, author of **Fat Chance: Beating the Odds Against Sugar, Processed Food, Obesity, and Disease** said *"The real problem is not in losing the weight but in keeping it off for any meaningful length of time. Numerous sources show that almost every lifestyle intervention works for the first three to six months. But then the weight comes rolling back."*

There are many confusing questions about obesity, losing weight and keeping it off:

- Why do we gain weight?
- Why is it easy for some of us and tough for others, especially T2 and pre-diabetics, to lose weight?
- Why weight loss comes back after a couple of months?

There are countless of theories out there talking about losing weight and keeping it off. Let's shed some lights on some of these assumptions.

1. Eat more and move less, make you gain weight. It is the most common mainstream belief.
2. Carbohydrates make you fat.
3. Fat makes you fat.
4. Fructose makes you fat.
5. Low carb high fat or Keto diet is the only way to lose weight.
6. Not all calories created equal.
7. Negative calories balance leads to weight loss.
8. High protein, low carb and low to medium natural fat is the best.
9. It is the quality, not the quantity of what you eat that controls your weight gain.
10. Fasting is the only solution.

Everyone is different

When it comes to weight management, regardless of the above different theories. There is no one system fits all. I know people that eat starches, sweet and fat like monsters, but they are actually underweight. By the way that doesn't mean they are healthy, remember the visceral fat! On the contrary, I know people like myself; can gain weight even with 30 grams a day of carbs. I am not kidding when I say, "even smelling the aroma of hot bread can make me fat!" In my case, eating a high carbohydrate diet makes gaining weight unbelievably fast, yet cutting carbs stabilizes my weight but it doesn't help me much in losing it. Ditto with high fat.

Gary Taubes explained this perfectly in his book <u>Why We Get Fat</u> when he talked about the car pedometer's fuel indicator example where Full petrol symbol is for (Fat) and Empty is for

(Energy). When it comes to metabolism, some people have their indicator points easily to the fat side, as an indication they tend to store a portion of what they eat as body fat instead of burning it by muscles and these are the overweight people. While some others have their indicator points, effortlessly, to the energy side (Empty). They have more energy to be burned in physical activities rather than store it as fat. These guys are lucky and don't gain weight easily.[57]

He explained that these "no-gain-weight guys" have their LPL (Lipoprotein Lipase) more active in their muscles cells and less active in their fat cells. Therefore, they can utilize fat for fuel and do not tend to store energy as fat. On the contrary, overweight fellows have their LPL very active on their fat cells (adipose tissues) and less active on their muscles cells, so they convert any extra energy to stored fat.

Another hormone plays a big role in making us fat is Leptin. Leptin is a hormone secreted by body fat cells. It tells our brain, there is enough fat stored in our fat cells and it is time to feel full and raise metabolism.

According to Dr. Robert Lustig, insulin contributes to obesity by blocking the leptin signal in the brain when the insulin level gets too high. When people become leptin resistant, their brain cannot read the message leptin wants to transmit. Therefore, continuous high levels of insulin might be one of the main reasons for leptin resistance and accordingly continuous hunger and endless weight gain.

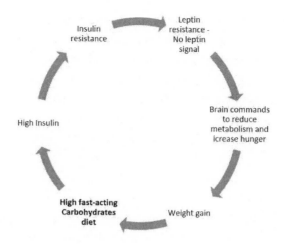

It was not shocking news to me to realize that both Insulin and Leptin are the two criminals prevented me from losing weight. As an insulin-dependent diabetic, I knew I could only lose weight when I reduce my total daily insulin units. However, this is not as easy as it sounds because insulin in my case (and in case of every insulin-dependent) is necessary. When I said reducing total daily insulin, I meant not only reducing my bolus units but also reducing my daily basal insulin units (DBIU) as well.

Let me give you an example; when my weight was 245 lb I was taking about 37 of DBIU, when my weight went down to 234 lb I was injecting 31 of DBIU and when I reach 225 lb, I was injecting around 28 DBIU. The more weight I lose the lesser total daily insulin (TDI) I take. But, again, I cannot lose weight unless I reduce my TDI further down and this is the big DILEMA and the vicious circle many people with diabetes have to deal with most of the time. **To lose weight you need to reduce the injected/secreted insulin and to reduce the injected/secreted insulin you need to lose weight!**

In fact, many insulin-dependent PWD especially T2 or LADA (they gain weight easier than T1) cannot lower their basal rate much; otherwise, their blood sugar numbers will hike. They are in an undeliberate fat storage mode all the time. Activating LPL, deactivating HSL, blocking Leptin, Lacking Amylin hormone, (unfortunately insulin-dependent PWD don't produce it) and provoking the Ghrelin hormone (the hunger hormone). Usually, these fellows are insensitive to insulin and are very sensitive to carbs at the same time. Therefore, any small amount of fast-acting carbohydrates will hike their weight up dramatically. I am one of those people.

Amylin is another hormone makes it hard for insulin-dependent to lose weight. The lack of amylin adds to the dilemma and makes controlling BS a hard mission. Beta cells in insulin-dependent don't produce amylin but they do produce glucagon which contributes to raising blood sugar by signaling the liver to decompose some of the glycogen to glucose and release it in the bloodstream. It seems harsh, I know!

Amylin mission is to delay stomach emptying after eating and reduce the liver production of glucose, so the blood sugar control becomes easier. It also suppresses the appetite, which keeps blood sugar stable between meals. The lack of amylin is one of the main reasons for the hardship of losing weight for the insulin-dependent diabetics.

How I broke the cycle

Initially, I tried the low carb WOE. My weight gain halted and my blood sugar normalized, but I did not lose weight. Then, I switched to the Low Carb/High Fat (LCHF) WOE. This WOE did not work for me either. I gained weight eating high or medium fat, even while eating very low carb.

At this point, I also added daily brisk walking for 1 hour. This improved my insulin sensitivity, which was beneficial, but no weight reduction occurred because of adding exercise.

By the way, there is a misconception among many people thinking that they can lose weight if they just exercise, no matter what they eat. Nothing could be further from the truth. This is a fallacy, and the truth is; you cannot lose weight by exercising while you eat the wrong food. Exercise will benefit in many other areas but not losing weight especially when you eat the wrong food. Dr. Robert Lustig said, *"Exercise is the single best thing you can do for yourself. It's way more important than dieting and easier to do. Exercise works at so many levels — except one: your weight."*

Regardless of any WOE I followed, if I just slacked a little bit for a week or two, my weight would creep up mercilessly. At first, I thought I could still include some fast-acting carb treats: a spoon of sugar in my coffee, a piece of fruit daily, one scoop of ice cream occasionally, a few French fries once biweekly. These seemingly small "cheats" resulted in an immediate weight gain and higher basal needs due to glycogen replenishment. I could not escape the fact of food increases my insulin intake.

Back in 2009, I was using pre-mixed insulin, which did nothing to control my blood sugar. Hence, I had a lot of wasted energy in the form of extra glucose roaming around my bloodstream and damaging my organs. My weight, at the time, was about 210 lb as compared to 240 lb when I used the right insulin and was able to control my blood sugar later on. That made sense to me. Weight crept up slowly in direct proportion to controlling blood sugar. This gave me a practical clue about the role of insulin in making us fat.

Carbohydrate intake provokes the secretion of insulin. Eating more fast-acting carbohydrates lead to more insulin production. In the end, this causes insulin and then leptin resistance making weight loss an illusion. Therefore, as a diabetic, I knew the first step had to come through dramatically reducing fast-acting carb consumption. This would accordingly, reduce insulin usage, which would lead to improving Leptin sensitivity as well.

Dr. David Perlmutter tells us in the <u>Grain Brain</u>, *"Leptin essentially controls mammalian metabolism. Most people think that this is the job of the thyroid but leptin actually controls the thyroid, which regulates the rate of metabolism."*[58]

I stuck to the low carb, medium protein, low to medium healthy fat WOE but with the amount of insulin I used, basal in specific, weight loss continued to be an impossible mission. But, at least I had stopped the weight gain.

Next, I discovered Dr. Jason Fung and Jimmy Moore's book The Complete Guide to Fasting. I read it very carefully. I weighed 246 lb when I implemented what I read in this great book.

I told myself "why not give it a shot". Therefore, I started fasting for 24 hours and re-fed one low carb meal, medium fat and protein per day, but still, nothing happened. I increased the fasting to 48 hours and re-fed. To my amazement, I showed some positive results and started losing weight. I extended the fasting to 72 hours and as result not only I lost weight but also I reduced my basal insulin about 30% the third day. So fasting for a bit longer periods caused double positive effects for me: eliminating my bolus insulin for a few days (while fasting) along with reducing my basal insulin, which what I exactly needed to lose weight as a very-weight-loss-resisting insulin-dependent diabetic.

I would also say, using Victoza, as per my doctor advice, helped me sometimes to control weight and blood sugar. Victoza is used by T2 diabetics but many doctors use it for T1. As you will see, it does some good job parallel to insulin work, which helps some T1 diabetics to control BS as well. Victoza does the same job as Symlin, which is a substitute for the amylin hormone. Both insulin and amylin are not produced any more by the insulin-dependent beta cells person.

Victoza slows emptying stomach, reduces the liver production of glucose, suppresses appetite, and let the pancreas secrete some insulin (hormone GLP-1 work). As you can see the first three functions supports both T1 and T2 while the fourth is for T2 only.

However, I always quit it for the side effect of vomiting feeling all the time. Victoza helps me a lot, when using, in stabilizing blood sugar as it reduced the liver production of glucose and with some crazy liver like mine with crazy dawn phenomenon, this means a lot. To give you a hint, using Victoza reduces my basal about 15 to 20% just because of the reducing-glucose-liver-effect.

Victoza works so well with me the first two weeks of starting using it. But, for some reason, it doesn't work efficiently (with me) after a couple of weeks of using. Anyway, it gives me a good launch at the beginning when needed. One more thing, the side effect written in Victoza pamphlet[59] is scary. One of them is pancreatitis! I do not use it much for this specific reason.

If you are diabetic and had tried everything to lose weight without success, I recommend you consider fasting and see what happens, of course, after discussing it with your physician. Be flexible with yourself while fasting. Start gradually. Do not be so strict on yourself and do 96 hours of fasting on your first fast! I believe this could be a fruitful approach for PWD with no hope of losing weight, like myself.

Fasting requires willpower and patience until your body adapts to it. You will eventually become accustomed to it. Fasting opens up a new avenue for people that appear resistant to weight loss. Again, I hate generalization. I cannot say there is one-way fits all, it all depends on the individual acceptance, responses, and results. However, I can only say, "you are the only one who can decide what is good and working for you and what is not". Results and results only, determine the worth of any intervention.

Chapter 19: Strong Young Man

"The more people overeat carbohydrates, the more they will become obese, even if they exercise a lot."

Dr. Richard K. Bernstein

I n January 2018, I posted on my diabetes FB page asking if anyone in Germany wanted a copy of my book <u>What You Do Not Know About Diabetes</u> written in Arabic. I announced that I would be traveling there in three days. I got a reply back from a young man called Tamer asking me, which German city did I plan to visit? I said, "Koln."

He replied "OMG What a coincidence, I live and study in Koln. Yes, please bring me a copy of your book as I am in great need of it."

The plan was to arrive early at the Frankfurt airport, take the train to Koln, take care of my business there, and then meet him in the evening at my hotel. It was a very cold December day in the adorable city of Koln. I finished my work around 7 pm as planned and tried to locate a low carb meal in Koln, but it was not an easy mission. The wheat culture there is prevalent. Anyway, I managed to eat some plain Shawerma (meat) in a hurry and headed back to the hotel, passing by the majestic Koln Cathedral, to meet Tamer.

Tamer came to the hotel at 8 pm as agreed. A tall young man with T1 diabetes (as he told me), with exhausted brown eyes. The paleness in his face reveals his uncontrolled blood sugar. He met me with a baby face smile that uncovered his beautiful soul. I could easily see that he had read a lot about diabetes management from my Facebook diabetes page and other pages. He is a Syrian young man who fled the country to escape the horrible war at the time. He came to Germany as a refugee, passing by many European countries that rejected refugees. He was hosted by a German family who took great care of him for eleven months. Staying with this family helped him to learn the German language so fast, which enabled him to start studying in the pre-medical school of Koln University in no time.

Three months after settling in Germany, he received the bad news of his father's death back home in Syria, which left his mother alone with his sister and brother. At that point, in his story, tears fell as he spoke and he kept silent for a moment. Among all these painful life events, he was diagnosed with T1 diabetes after suffering all the well-known symptoms of thirst, frequent urination, and exhaustion. The diagnosis came right after two major events in his life. First, he left the comfortable life with the German family home to a rented room in a city that was located 60 km away from the university, so he could afford the rent, just days before he received the news of his father's passing. Second, two months later, his mother was diagnosed with heart disease and was scheduled for emergency surgery. Tamer got a part-time job to save some money and send it to his mother so she could afford to have the required surgery.

Through all of this, he forgot about his diabetes and his BS numbers were all over the place. Apparently, he followed the same mainstream advice we all know very well. Eat high carbs, low fat, inject fixed industrial doses of fast-acting insulin and eat to cover it. Then, he was switched to pre-mixed insulin with no hope for achieving normal blood sugar. While telling me his story, his body movement revealed frustration, depression, and hopelessness. I felt that my short presence refreshed his sad family memories again, which made me feel guilty. However, after telling his story, he looked more comfortable and released. Being a relief for some of his stress and agony, made me happy.

He got his copy of my book and handed me a copy of the German language version of the great book Grain Brain. I have no clue about the German language, but I was delighted by such a gesture of appreciation from a wonderful young man. We spoke a long time about diabetes management and covered all issues about insulin, factors, injection timing, normal blood sugar numbers and reducing carbohydrates consumption. That was Monday; he left at 11 pm promising that we will meet again in BON on Wednesday right after I finish my work.

On Wednesday, we met at 3 pm and walked around about three hours in the charming old city of BON, surrounded by a magical environment of tourists and a freezing zero degree temperature. We visited Beethoven's house and the old city. We ate lunch together. To my surprise, he had read almost half the book in two days. He asked me many questions about food, low carbohydrates substitutes, recipes, and insulin, etc. I felt so proud of this strong young man while answering his questions. It was an honor to know him. Tamer's perseverance and endurance made me feel that all my problems are trivial and indeed blessings compared to his struggles.

My flight back home was at midnight. After an emotional good-bye, Tamer did not let his sight off me until I disappeared into the train taking me to the Frankfurt airport! The train remained five more minutes at Koln station. As the train sped up leaving the station, I spotted Tamer sitting comfortably on one of the station's seats while passionately reading the book! That moment, I strongly realized that this young man would be something big one day.

Now after one year, he is an expert in diabetes management with a pump, CGM, and flat blood sugar profile. Every couple of weeks he sends me some amazing pictures of low carb plates he cooks himself. He is no longer eating starches or sugar. And, guess what?

He enjoys normal blood sugar all the time (see his CGM picture below) and his recent HbA1c was 4.8% instead of 10%. It is an honor to know you, Tamer, really.

Chapter 20: My story with insulin pump

"You can improve insulin sensitivity and reduce your risk of diabetes (not to mention all manner of brain diseases) simply by making lifestyle changes that melt that fat away. And if you add exercise to the dieting, you'll stand to gain even bigger benefits."

Dr. David Perlmutter.

I never thought of using the insulin pump for two reasons; **first,** I did not admire constant apparatus attachment. **Second**, my health insurance doesn't cover insulin pump and its accessories. Four years ago, Insulin pump's initial cost was around $8200 and the monthly spending is about $1000. This is doubtlessly expensive. Therefore, I always postponed the decision to get it.

Admittedly, one of the major reasons encouraged me to change my decision was the dawn phenomenon. However, somehow, I managed to control it with the MDI approach but it wasn't the perfect control I was aiming for. I desperately wanted something that could divide my basal needs throughout the day to multiple and different levels of dosing.

In fact, my basal need fluctuates severely in the twenty-four hours period. That made it hard to control my blood sugar with one dose or even split dose of basal over the twenty-four hours. When

I used the freestyle libre (a flash glucose monitoring) I realized that my afternoon basal unit-per-hour was (and still is) almost one-third my nighttime basal unit-per-hour need! This explained why, sometimes, I would get afternoon hypoglycemia and sleeping time hyperglycemia using fixed MDI basal injection (twice a day).

To make a long story short, four years ago I decided to purchase my first Medtronic pump, model 754 Veo pump. I took a month to precisely tweak the right basal rates for myself. This confirmed my basal hourly rate of two units/hour from midnight to 9 am, 0.7 unit/hour from 11 am to 9 pm and around 1.4 units/hour other times. That, itself, solved my dawn phenomenon dilemma once and for all. To be honest, if this was the only advantage of the insulin pump, it would be enough to condone all other disadvantages.

The insulin pump pros

1. Its priceless ability to be set for different levels of basal throughout a twenty-four hours period. This helps PWD who suffer from severe dawn phenomenon like myself.

2. The square wave bolus option is one of the greatest pump advantages. It enables you to distribute your bolus needs in an hour or more to cover protein or very slow-acting carbohydrate.

3. The ability to inject a tiny dose of bolus with decimals makes the pump a great deal for T1 children, considering their high sensitivity to insulin. I know a T1 two-year-old kid who has a correction factor of 200 mg/dl, i.e. one unit of FAI brings his blood sugar down 200 mg/dl. Imagine if his blood sugar is 130 mg/dl and want to reduce it to 100 mg/dl, it will be almost a mission impossible without insulin dilution or an insulin pump. Pump minimum bolus can reach 0.025 units. In this kid case, he can easily get 0.15 units and he will reach his goal with no fear of hypoglycemia. This is a magnificent advantage indeed.

4. The ease of recording the IC ratio and correction factor makes it easy for many mothers to manage their T1 kids' meals insulin and correction needs.

5. Calculation IOB is a valuable advantage as well; as it makes you extra cautious when you intend to inject insulin twice within three hours.

6. One of the greatest advantages of the insulin pump is being able to set temporary basal or even cut the basal for a while for any reason. I use this feature when I feel I am approaching hypoglycemia and before exercise.

The insulin pumps cons

1. From day one, my body never accepted the infusion set material (Teflon). It causes inflammation on the insertion site after less than 8 hours of inserting it. The insertion site gets red and inflamed all the time. I have tried everything including proper hygiene, but the problem persists. I googled it a bit and found out many people shared the same problem. They advised me to use a metal infusion set instead, which I did, by using a "Sure T" set. This is definitely better, but still, I have to change the insertion location every day. By the way, I also confirmed this is not happening because of adhesive irritation.

2. I have never managed to bolus more than two units at once, without the insertion spot getting inflamed, bumpy and painful. Therefore, I use the insulin pump as a basal tool only and I bolus by Novorapid pen all the time.

3. I get scars constantly, so rotation is so important for proper absorption of insulin. Dr. Bernstein talked about the scars issue as a major disadvantage of the insulin pump.

4. Freedom is compromised; there is no better feeling than being unattached. You feel free to swim, shower, sleep, run and pass through airport security scanner any time without

thinking of the thing attached to you. I cannot deny this big mental effect.

The upshot is that the advantages of insulin pump outweigh its disadvantages. The basal adjustment's advantage is priceless. Perhaps, the peace of being able to inject a very tiny amount of insulin for your T1 diabetic baby would be your best advantage. Maybe the best advantage for someone else is the peace of having all factors and IOB stored in his/her pump. In the end, it works fine with me combined with three months a year of MDI to rest and feel the freedom. To be honest, I value freedom so much; this is why I am back to MDI now!

Chapter 21: high carbs vs normal blood sugar

"Breakfast: The most important meal to skip."
Dr. Jason Fung.

The uncertainty is the enemy of achieving normal blood sugar. After many years of adhering to the mainstream guidelines and following the high carbs WOE, it was a no brainer to find out that it is impossible to normalize blood sugar while eating high carb foods. Matching high carbs food with insulin is an impossible mission filled with inevitable uncertainty. And, the uncertainty is the enemy of control. I am not talking about the control of HbA1c of 6 or above which is possible with a bit higher percentage of carbs, but this is not the real control I am looking for. I am talking about the achievement of normal blood sugar of HbA1c below 5.5.

Generally speaking, I followed the ADA guidelines of 45 to 60 grams of carbs a meal for about seven years. While living the high carbs life, I tried every possible way to get the required BS control. I mastered MDI techniques, learned all the factors (IC ratio, correction factor, insulin on board calculations), understood glycemic index and glycemic load, mastered correct timing of injections, close prediction of different foods' digestion patterns, and I became a professional in carb counting. Unfortunately, none of these efforts got me closer to normal blood sugar. It was futile.

Why was it impossible to achieve normal blood sugar while eating this way? Before I delve further into my answer, let me share a piece of Dr. William Davis's book <u>Wheat Belly</u>. He said it perfectly, "*Years ago I used ADA diet in treating diabetic patients. Following the carbohydrate intake advice of the ADA, I watched patients gain weight, experience deteriorating blood glucose control, increase need for medication, and develop diabetes complications. The ADA advises people with diabetes to cut fat, reduce saturated fat and include 45 to 60 grams of carbohydrate–preferably healthy whole wheat–in each meal or 135 to 180 grams of carbohydrate per day, not including snacks. It is in essence, a fat-phobic, carbohydrate-centered diet, with 55 to 65 percent of calories from carbohydrates. If I were to sum up the views of the ADA towards diet, it would be: Go ahead and eat sugar and foods that increase blood sugar, just be sure to adjust your medication to compensate*"[60].*

Now let's discuss the discernible factors that make it impossible to control blood sugar while eating this amount of daily carbohydrates:

1. One gram of carbohydrate raises the blood sugar of 150 lb non-obese T1 diabetic around 5 to 6 mg/dl.[61] If he follows the ADA guidelines and eats around 180 grams of carbs daily, i.e. 60 grams of carbs per meal. These 60 grams of carbohydrates will rapidly raise his BS 300 to 360 mg/dl, which is a flood of glucose in his bloodstream. No insulin will catch or match such high and quickly elevated blood sugar.

2. Any mistake in carbohydrates counting will lead to extra or less insulin injected. This mistake could be due to less experience, hidden carbohydrates in the meal or wrong labeling. Dr. Bernstein mentioned in his book that food producers are permitted a margin of error of ±20% deviated from their labeling of ingredients. In the case of 60 grams of carbs per meal, this 20% will lead to

an uncertainty of ±12 grams of carbohydrates (60 * 20%). Multiply this by 5 mg/dl. The result will be an uncertainty of ±60 mg/dl in this man BS after eating. Therefore, if his BS was 100 mg/dl before food and injected equivalent units of insulin to the 60 grams of carbohydrates in his meal in order to reach 100 mg/dl again after food, this uncertainty will affect his BS result with ±60 mg/dl. Therefore, instead of being 100 mg/dl after food, his BS will probably be either 160 or 40 mg/dl (100 ± 60). Imagine, if you eat more than 60 grams of carbs in one meal, what will happen then?[62]

3. With such amount of carbohydrates, any miscalculation in IC ratio (Insulin to carbs ratio) makes a huge mistake that will show itself via highs or lows of BS measurements after food.

4. If fast-acting insulin is injected a long time prior to eating and food digested was delayed, your BS will drop then will rise again. In other words, you will go through hypoglycemia and then hyperglycemia.

5. If you inject fast-acting insulin closer to eating time and food was digested faster than expected, then BS will rise first then perhaps hypoglycemia will occur later.

6. The higher the dose of insulin, the higher the uncertainty and the higher the loss in injected insulin units. This happens due to the immune system attack against big doses of insulin as per the law of insulin absorption by Dr. Richard Bernstein.[63] The 150 lb person has an insulin correction factor of about 40 mg/dl (i.e. one fast-acting insulin unit lowers his BS about 40 mg/dl). For the 60 grams of carbs eaten, he requires 60÷5=12 units (assuming his IC ratio is 5). As per Dr. Bernstein, the uncertainty reaches 29% of the injected units in such large dose. i.e. 12 x 29% = 3.48 units, rounded to four uncertain units of insulin. So out of the

12 units of insulin injected; only eight units will be effective and the remaining four (or part of them) are destroyed by the immune system. This will create 4 x 40 = 160 mg/dl of uncertainty in BS expectations. So if you expect your BS to be 100 after eating it may reach to 100+160 = 260 mg/dl. As Dr. Bernstein said, "*The result is totally haphazard blood sugars and complete unpredictability, just by the virtue of the varying amount of insulin absorbed*".[64] Now imagine if the same person ate a low carb meal, the injected insulin should be much less and there will be almost no uncertainty.

7. Uncontrolled diabetes causes gastroparesis as one of the complications. It means unpredictable digestion pattern. Consuming high carbohydrates meals, while gastroparesis exists, means you want to match FAI with unknown digestion pattern, which is impossible and will get the blood sugar profile out of control.

8. If IOB (Insulin On Board) is miscalculated, you will see problems with BS after eating, either higher or lower than expected. This is a big problem, especially if the injected dose is high. For example, the IOB for three units of injected fast-acting insulin at the beginning of the third hour is only one unit, compared to IOB of six units for 18 units of fast-acting insulin injected. **So the higher the carbs content in your meal, the higher the insulin dose, the higher the IOB in the third hour and the difficult the guesswork, if correction needed at the third hour.**

9. According to Dr. Bernstein law of small numbers: "Big inputs make big mistakes, small inputs make small mistakes".[65] In other words, the smaller the carbohydrate content in a meal, the smaller the fast-acting insulin dose required, the smaller the expected mistakes and the easier to fix them. Conversely, the

higher the carbohydrate content in a meal, the larger the fast-acting insulin dose required, the bigger the expected mistakes and the harder to fix them. Mistakes here means mistakes in guesswork, miscalculating injection timing in related to a meal, wrong carbs counting, digestion expectations, IOB calculation, wrong consideration of IC ratio, etc.

10. The higher the BS will reach, the harder it is to bring it down, as insulin behaves differently when blood sugar is high. When BS rises, your body cells try to stop insulin from pushing extra toxic glucose into them, via making their insulin receptors resistant to insulin. Therefore, when your BS is 190 mg/dl and you want to get it down to 90 mg/dl, you will definitely use higher correction factor than if you are 120 and wants to get it down to 90 mg/dl. Myself I experienced this phenomenon many times in the era of my high carbs WOE.

If you are T1, T2 or even non-diabetic eating high carbohydrate diet and doubting what I mentioned, I invite you to do the following experiment. Forget about measuring your BS two hours after a meal. Instead, for the next couple of days, measure your BS 30, 45, 60 and 75 minutes after eating high fast-acting carbohydrate food and use your insulin maneuverability skills then see for yourself what your BS numbers will be. The following couple of days, do the same thing but with low carb food. You are the judge.

Chapter 22: A Diabetic in the surgery room

"Like many young doctors, I had received virtually no instruction in nutrition. Then, as now, medical schools focused almost exclusively on drugs and surgery, even though lifestyle causes most cases of heart disease and other chronic disabling conditions."
Dr. David Ludwig

I t is time. Tuesday, November 24th, 2015 at 11 am, I had just arrived at the hospital and getting ready to be admitted for knee surgery after 9 months of continuous pain due to a meniscus tear in my right knee. The nurse prepared me for the 1:00 pm surgery and a little conversation with her went as follows:

"I am a T1 diabetic and I definitely want no intravenous glucose to be given to me while I am half-asleep in operation," I said.

"Sir; the doctor will decide this, not the patient. Anyway, I believe it is a protocol that must be followed and it cannot be changed unless the specialist says so," Nurse said.

"No, it can be changed, and I already agreed with my surgeon to put me on a non-lactated saline solution, if required. It is just a 40 minutes surgery and I insist," I said.

She called the nursing supervisor who came and started to argue with me as well. Then he noticed the insulin pump on me and asked, "What is this?"

I said, "Insulin pump,".

"Insulin pump!" Supervisor replied.

"Yes, insulin pump," I replied.

"What kind of insulin do you use in it?" Supervisor asked.

"Novorapid," I replied.

"I think you will have to take it off during the surgery," Supervisor replied.

"No, I do not have to. It gives me my body need for basal insulin. Anyway, I will discuss this with the surgeon," I replied. The room was suddenly filled with four nurses listening.

"Even basal insulin only, you will have to take the pump off sir," Supervisor replied.

"No, I will not. Because, again, it is my basal insulin instrument," I replied.

"What is basal insulin?" Another nurse asked.

"It is the insulin required to match the glucose secreted from the liver to serve all involuntary movement's energy requirement of my internal organs inside my body. Basal insulin makes sure that energy is available for digestion, breathing, heart pumping, kidney filtration, etc.," I replied.

"Sir, you are so inclined in medical information, how do you learn all of this?" Another nurse asked.

"Well, I am an educated insulin-dependent diabetic who learned how to take very good care of his own version of diabetes, I had no other choice," I replied.

It is time for the anesthesia to be injected. At the same time, another nurse measured my blood sugar, and it was 84 mg/dl. She reported it to the surgeon who was shocked and said, "You are hypoglycemic, please eat some sweet or drink some juice to raise up your BS before we start. It is accepted to be higher than that, so why to take the risk!"

"This is a normal blood sugar range doctor," I said. "Moreover the precise basal adjustment in my pump guarantees that this will be almost a steady number as long as I am fasting as requested before this surgery," I explained.

They called the hospital endo who shows his irritation about the number 84 mg/dl and I convinced him that my basal insulin is well adjusted and I will not go hypo because of the following reasons:

1. Enlite sensor is on and it will cut off the basal immediately if any hypo happens.
2. I am fasting, so the sensor reading should be very close to real BS reading.
3. There will be no bolus to cause any hypo.
4. I have not had a single hypoglycemic episode for a long time since I started on a Low Carbohydrate diet.
5. I am following the law of small numbers of Dr. Richard Bernstein, which minimizes the chance of hypoglycemia occurrence.
6. To make you happy, I will reduce 10% of the basal insulin for the next one hour.

The Endo looked at the surgeon and said, "Fine, looks like he knows what he is doing. It's OK for me. You can go ahead and start the procedure."

I finished the 40 minutes operation peacefully with no glucose needed (only non-lactated Saline as I requested). My pump was on and my BS was between 80 and 90 during the surgery.

The whole day after the surgery, I was talking about diabetes management with some nursing staff who were eager to learn more. I was also happy to have the chance to spread the word again and again.

In one of Dr. Bernstein's Diabetes University's videos,[66] Dr. Bernstein told a true story of a T1 girl who was hospitalized for a vomiting illness. In the emergency room, they wanted to give her intravenous glucose and her father argued and refused. He spoke to Dr. Bernstein on the phone and asked him to speak with the director of the pediatric emergency who is insisting on the glucose drip. During the phone conversation, Dr. Bernstein learned that the director wanted to give the T1 diabetic girl 250 ml of D10 (10% dextrose) for at least four hours as per the hospital policy.

Dr. Bernstein asked her "Do you have any idea how much this amount of glucose would raise her blood sugar?"

She said "no!"

Dr. Bernstein did the math and figured out that this much of glucose will raise her BS to about 2000 mg/dl (she was 90 mg/dl)!

Dr. Bernstein asked the director "What is the death rate for T1 kids with Ketoacidosis in your hospital?"

She replied "55%."

"So you want to give this little girl a likelihood of 55% of dying when, right now, the only problem is that she is vomiting?!" said Dr. Bernstein.

"This is the hospital rules," she answered.

"What if you write in the chart that you spoke to the child's physician and he said that she couldn't have intravenous glucose? Would that get you off the hook?" Dr. Bernstein asked.

"Yes," she said.

This scary story is real and it reveals how serious it could be for T1 diabetics under the mercy of hospitals' rules and under the mercy of a physician who knows little about diabetes.

Moral of the story: As Dr. Bernstein said, *"If you want to control your blood sugar you must know about diabetes just like your physician does,"* and I add, *"You must know about your diabetes more than your physician does."*

Chapter 23: World champion of Triglyceride

*"Eating high-cholesterol foods has no impact on our actual
cholesterol levels, and the alleged correlation between higher
cholesterol and higher cardiac risk is an absolute fallacy."*
Dr. David Perlmutter

About five years prior to being diagnosed with diabetes, I
found out that my lipid profile was ominous with an
outrageous triglyceride (TG) level. My TG level was between 700 to
1000 mg/dl (recommended < 100 mg/dl) and reaching as insanely
as 1200 mg/dl at times! When the number was that high, the lab
always stamped my report with a special stamp: "the results have
been repeatedly confirmed." My LDL was high, My HDL was low
and my total cholesterol was about 300 mg/dl while it is
recommended, by mainstream organizations, to be under 200
mg/dl.

My physician, unarguably, prescribed me statins and a TG
reducing drug. He was literally following current clinical
guidelines, which are endorsed by many of the large organizations.
I blindly followed his advice and used both medication for about 8
years. With my subsequent diabetes diagnosis, I had the chance to
read many books about diabetes, cholesterol management, and
nutrition science. Fortunately, this opportunity changed the way I

look at cholesterol. I gained a fresh perspective on the benefits of cholesterol and the damaging effects of statins.

Cholesterol (CHL)

I learned that CHL is not a harming substance to our bodies as commonly thought. Conversely, it is so beneficial to our bodies and to our brains specifically. CHL is a vital substance that greatly needed to perform many crucial functions in our bodies such as:

- CHL plays a big role in creating Vitamin D with sun exposure.
- CHL is a major factor in forming many hormones like Cortisol, Estrogen, and Testosterone.
- CHL is found in our cells structures. Cell membranes are made of CHL to guarantee fluidity and permeability. So, cells can only allow some substances or molecules such as glucose, for example, to pass through the membrane from the outside to the inside and not vice versa.
- CHL helps in forming the Bile liquid with the aid of the liver in the gallbladder, which helps in fat digestion.
- Many studies show that people with cognitive diseases like Alzheimer, Schizophrenia, ADHD, Dementia, and autism are found to have less CHL in their brains. Other studies tell us that a high percentage of CHL in the elderly has a significant connection with less mortality and better health.[67] Dr. Perlmutter wrote about this in details in his book Grain Brain.

There is no such thing of good CHL and bad CH. It is all about carriers of the CHL, whether or not these carriers have been glycated. The glycation of the carriers is the biggest determinant. LDL, the so-called bad CHL, is a lipoprotein, not a cholesterol. It actually carries CHL to the brain along with fatty acids and antioxidants. This is one of the reasons why statins are so bad for you. It severely diminishes the number of LDL particles and accordingly, reduces the CHL, fatty acids and antioxidants reaching the brain. This causes many cognitive functions issues especially memory issues. It is not uncommon for people prescribed statins to suffer from extreme forgetfulness. Many times, when I was taking statins, I would put things down and not be able to remember where I put them five minutes later. More information about statins can be found in Dr. Duane Graveline's books The Dark Side of Statins and Lipitor The Memory Thief.

Glycation

When blood sugar elevates, the glucose molecules will bind to blood proteins. LDL and HDL are partial blood proteins. In fact, they are lipoproteins (fat and protein) so that CHL, as a fat substance, could dissolve in the fat part of the lipoprotein while the protein part dissolves in the bloodstream and move freely to transfer the CHL to various parts of the body. When glycation happens, glucose binds to the protein part of the lipoprotein and causes glycated LDL and glycated HDL. Of course, PWD (with uncontrolled BS) are the most group of people that their blood proteins are more prone to be glycated, because of the ongoing possibility of high blood sugar. And that explains the high rate of coronary heart diseases, strokes and nerves damage among PWD with uncontrolled BS.

Glycation could be reversible if we normalize blood sugar. Otherwise, the glycated protein will form advanced glycated end-products (AGEs) which speeds up all harmful processes inside our bodies. These are the processes known as oxidation and the formation of free radicals. AGEs from different glycated proteins link together in a process called cross-linking and causes even larger damage to our internal organs. Cross-linking adversely affects all body cells and put the body into an inflammatory state. One of the problems Cross-linking of AGEs causes is to increase the stiffness of the body's tissues such as arteries, bones (collagen) and muscles.[68] It also causes plaque deposition on the interior walls of arteries and ultimately causes atherosclerosis.

As we now see, the problem is not the good CHL or the bad one. It is all about high blood sugar that binds to proteins and forms glycated protein. I have learned that glycated proteins behave differently from non-glycated proteins. Glycation changes the chemical structure and functions of the glycated protein. Instead of being useful, they become harmful as it upregulates the inflammatory state in the body. Dr. Perlmutter said in Grain Brain, *"These days, more and more people are beginning to understand that coronary artery disease, a leading cause of heart attack, may actually have more to do with inflammation that it does with high cholesterol. This explains why aspirin, in addition to its blood-thinning properties, is useful in reducing risk not only for heart attacks but also for strokes."*[69] I could simply say that keeping a normal blood sugar will save your heart, nerves, brain and, arteries a big headache.

Our liver produces 75% of the CHL we measure in the lab, while the other 25% comes from what we eat. The less CHL we eat, the more our liver produces CHL and vice versa. Briefly, the less fat you eat, the more fat your liver will produce and accumulate. For this reason, the low fat diet does not work in reducing elevated CHL or elevated TG. I definitely witnessed that myself in my case.

Higher LDL level doesn't scare me anymore as long as I eat right. I learned that the type of LDL is so important in deciding the harmful effect of elevated LDL. LDL particles could be buoyant and large or small and dense. The small and dense particles are the problematic ones. They are the ones that love to stick to the internal walls of arteries, forming plaque and causes atherosclerosis later on.[70] Eating high a carb low fat diet causes the formation of the small and dense LDL. Eating low carb, healthy fat lead to the formation of buoyant and large LDL particles. They are the friendly ones that cause no damage. I make sure that my LDL particles are of the right type by eating right, fasting, and exercise.

146

Triglyceride (TG)

The most important thing I learned, was that the main culprit of high triglyceride level was eating an excess amount of fast-acting carbohydrates such as starches, wheat products, and fructose. Fructose in specific raises TG, as it has no digestion path and it goes directly from small intestines to the liver and gets converted to TG. The learning shifted my paradigm about lipid profile. Therefore, I started searching more how could I reduce my high TG numbers naturally?

Before I could naturally control my lipid profile, my TG reading was between 600 to 1200 mg/dl. My CHL was around 300 to 350 mg/dl, my HDL was between 29 to 33 mg/dl and LDL was 200 mg/dl or more. My physician had no choice but to put me on a double dose of TG reduction medicine and Statins for life. After a couple of months of taking TG medication, I could only get my TG number down to around 300 mg/dl. I was on this pattern for almost 8 years. I was stifled with the severe side effects of the medication such as muscle pain and memory loss. By extensive search, I figured out the negative effect of starches, fructose on the elevation of TG level, especially for people who own a compromised metabolism like myself. Then, I thought; let me eliminate the food raises my TG for a while, stop the medication, and see what happens?

To be honest, my physician warned me not to do that. He declined the idea that I would ever be able to lower my high TG number with food choices, especially with such extreme numbers. However, I have always believed that good choices make a difference in almost everything. And, it was worth the risk indeed. That was back in 2012.

I stopped the medication and immediately eliminated all bread, pasta, rice, fruits, potatoes, sugar, fructose, HFCS, honey and all starchy vegetables. I followed this WOE religiously along with periodical intermittent fasting for four months. Guess WHAT! My first TG lab work came with a number that I never have seen before:

159 mg/dl without medication. WOW! It astonished my physician and I was extremely joyful to get such a great result. I never even got close to this number despite using a double dose of TG reducing drug! Four more months of sticking to Low Carb, medium protein and medium healthy fat along with twice weekly of 24 hours intermittent fasting and BOOOOM my next reading of TG was 99 mg/dl. I know I lost the TG championship title, but I gained my health back!

To make sure the food I restrained was the real culprit. Every time I slacked and admitted some fructose and starches to my meals, my TG numbers hiked up again to the 300 or 400s in less than 7 days of doing so. It was not a secret that elevated TG has a direct relationship with Coronary Heart Disease (CHD). Elevated TG and low HDL are far more serious indicators for the occurrence of coronary heart diseases (CHD) than CHL or LDL. Maria Emmerich mentioned in her book <u>Keto-Adapted</u> that one of the major indicators to rely on is your TG/HDL ratio. If **TG/HDL = one** then you are in the ideal range and if it is less than two, means that you are still in a safe range.[71]

Normal TG helps in achieving normal blood sugar. I found that normal TG numbers dramatically helped me improve my insulin sensitivity. This finding is valid with many people with diabetes who suffer from elevated TG. The moment they control their TG, their insulin sensitivity is enhanced which helped them to get closer to normal blood sugar. In fact, elevated TG level indicates a higher risk of heart attack and death in men and women.[72]

One last thing about statin. Research by an Iowa State University scientist suggests that cholesterol-reducing drugs known as statins may lessen brain function. Dr. Yeon-Kyun Shin, a biophysics professor in the department of biochemistry, biophysics and molecular biology, says, "*If you deprive cholesterol from the brain, then you directly affect the machinery that triggers the release of neurotransmitters," said Shin. "Neurotransmitters affect the data-*

processing and memory functions. In other words -- how smart you are and how well you remember things."[73]

Next time your physician prescribes you statins or TG reducing drug, please think twice before taking it.

Chapter 24: Is it time to look for another physician

"It is unreasonable to expect medical doctors and pharmaceutical companies to tell you how to avoid their services by trying the alternatives."
Andrew Saul.

L iving with diabetes is so frustrating. It requires 24 X 7 X 365 attention. However, aiming for normal blood sugar should be your ultimate goal. You need to focus on the approaches that get you closer to your goal. One major approach is finding the right physician. You should search for a physician who believes in the importance of normalizing blood sugar for people with diabetes. In the meantime, you need to drift away from main-streamers who believe HbA1c of 6.5 or 7 is just fine. In brief, never follow any advice of any type that deviates from achieving your goal.

I received a message from a mother of 3-year-old T1 child saying that she visited almost all doctors in her city and all of them refused the low carb WOE for her T1 kid. Despite his BS profile that swings from 50 mg/dl to 300 mg/dl on a daily basis but they still refuse to get out of the old box to save the future of this unfortunate child. Another message from a wife with an attached picture of her diabetic husband's foot wound. The foot is about to be amputated because of a deep and horrible wound that doesn't respond to treatment. It gets worse despite tons of antibiotics and wound treatment. His doctor insisted to keep him on sulfonylureas for years, while his BS remained high all the time. Not one physician tried seriously to support him in controlling his BS (by insulin for example). He keeps on eating starches, sugar, and not one physician told him how important normalizing his blood sugar for his wound healing. They said, "This is diabetes." It is a real tragedy when people put their trust in their physicians and betrayed that way. This is why I always say (and remind myself) not to settle for less with diabetes because diabetes never settles for less if you do.

Do not make my mistake of sticking to a physician who believes you will deteriorate anyway, just because you are diabetic. Through years of experience in dealing with physicians, I have gathered some alarming signs. You should always remain alert for these signs when dealing with your physician. If he/she has advised you on one or more of the below list, then please do yourself a big favor and walk away unless you are ok with mediocre diabetes control and its consequences. Otherwise, look for another physician immediately. A physician who should support you in achieving your goal. I would like to call these signs "the danger signs."

When to walk away from your physician

1. Your physician prescribes you fixed doses of fast-acting insulin (FAI) and recommends that you eat a large amount of starches to cover these units. People with T1 diabetes should inject FAI according to what they eat and never eat to cover fixed doses of fast-acting insulin. By the way, this practice is very common in many countries.

2. Your physician still preaches about the harms of eggs and healthy fat, while he has no issue with bread, rice, juice, and pasta!

3. Your physician has no clue about the effect of fast-acting carbohydrate on your blood sugar and continues to talk to you in the "calories" language instead of "grams of carbohydrates" language.
4. Your physician tells you HbA1c of 6.5 is great and acceptable.
5. If your physician believes that HbA1c below 6.4% is dangerous and always refers to two studies ADVANCE and ACCORD, please walk away. For your information, these two studies were published in 2008. Briefly, they indicate that PWD who achieve HbA1c of 6.4% are slightly more prone to die from heart attacks than PWD with higher HbA1c. This is completely non-sense. It is especially important to note that 91.7% of the participant subjects in the ACCORD study were using Avandia or Actos drugs. Both drugs are very famous for causing heart attacks. While they found no difference in heart attack rates between the 6.4% HbA1c group and the higher HbA1c group in the ADVANCE study, most participants in 6.4% group used sulfonylureas drug (gliclazide) which is a safer drug compared to Avandia.[74] Moreover, in both studies, they consider an HbA1c of 6.4% is a tight control, which is not indeed. Such high HbA1c reveals a blood sugar average of 151 mg/dl, which is definitely high. If this HbA1c is sustained, you should anticipate bad complications to happen. **Therefore, if your physician believes you should have an HbA1c above 6.4% to avoid a heart attack rather than keeping a normal HbA1C under 5.5, please walk away immediately and look for someone who talks logic**.
6. Your physician starts you immediately on sulfonylureas (SN) as a newly diagnosed T2. People with T2 diabetes mainly suffer from insulin resistance and SN pushes their exhausted beta cells to secrete more insulin. The rational approach is to enhance insulin sensitivity by the proper

dietary approach, metformin, insulin sensitizers medication, and exercise (this is the initial approach of Dr. Bernstein).

7. Your doctor prescribes you a Statin for a minimal elevation of your cholesterol and advises you to follow a low fat high carb diet rather than recommending you, first, to cut starches, fructose, sugar and trans fat.

8. Your doctor puts you on pre-mixed insulin. With that, you lose both control and flexibility and you can never achieve normal BS.

9. You ask your physician about your insulin factors (IC ratio, correction factor, insulin on board) and he has no clue about them.

10. Your doctor advises you to keep the blood sugar of your child with T1 diabetes high to avoid hypoglycemia. Many physicians ask parents to keep their T1 kid's blood sugar around 200 mg/dl before sleeping to avoid hypoglycemia instead of fine-tuning their food and insulin needs to achieve normal BS. Of course, this will have devastating consequences on them in the future.

11. Your physician tells you that young kids with T1 diabetes don't get diabetes complications! Yes, I know many parents that had been told this by their physicians to justify keeping T1 kids on high BS, being afraid of hypoglycemia.

12. Your physician says that whole-wheat is good for you and won't raise your BS.

13. Your physician is a person with diabetes and can't control his own diabetes.

Watch out for these danger signs and make an informative and immediate move to find another physician before it is too late. These kidneys, nerves, heart, arteries and eyes belong to you and not anyone else. It is your responsibility to keep them healthy and away from damaging complications. Your blood sugar numbers should be the measure of any advice you receive from your doctor.

Remember, normalizing your blood sugar is an informed decision, only you shall make. Be sure to choose the physician who supports you on your goal.

Chapter 25: A message from a mother of T1 diabetic girl, by Carol Friend

"The bottom line is pretty irrefutable: What good for the heart is good for the brain."
Rudolph Tanzi and Ann Parson, from Good Calories Bad Calories, Gary Taubes

Nearing the end of 2018, as this book was in its final editing, the NIH requested public commentary on the draft of the Nutrition Research Plan for the upcoming year. Details can be found here: https://www.niddk.nih.gov/about-niddk/strategic-plans-reports/strategic-plan-nih-nutrition-research I would like to share my response with you:

I am neither a doctor nor a nutrition researcher, but the past and future decisions of the NIH impact my life directly. First and foremost, I am a mother. My daughter has Type 1 diabetes. I, myself, have T2 diabetes and am a health care professional by trade. I am specific in that order because it is the former aspect of my life that brought me against my will into the world of diabetes and the mire that has become nutrition research.

My daughter was diagnosed with diabetes at the age of two. As is typical of very small children, control of her blood sugar was nightmarishly difficult despite the very best care, following the very best available clinical guidelines. Eventually, on the pump, we were able to achieve HbA1c around 7.5 and a level of control which was deemed PDG (pretty darn good) for her then age of five. However, she continued to fluctuate dramatically throughout the day and night. And, at this level of control, she went on to develop gastroparesis. As a healthcare professional, I knew that the complications would only continue to accrue and she was only in the 1st grade. There had to be a better way.

Indeed, there was. I found Dr. Bernstein's Diabetes Solution. At first glance, it sounded heretical and not unlike snake oil. I put myself on the regimen and lost 40 lbs. We took Sadie to him, transitioned off the pump and within days we stepped into the eye of the storm. After years of being spun around the periphery at the mercy of the disease, we were immediately inside an eerie calm. Her HbA1Cs remained between 5.8 and 6.0 without difficulty. Her constant nausea and burgeoning anxiety virtually disappeared. I was astounded.

However, though I stood calm and protected in the eye of the storm, I was forced to watch others still struggling in the powerful whirlwind. Clinical guidelines seemed to set in concrete despite the dismal control they afforded. In addition, we were separated from other children with diabetes by our dramatic difference in the regimen.

What is that you are saying? "I am glad you found something that works for you." I have heard this more times than I can count.

Well, now after our 18 years journey with T1 diabetes, we are no longer alone. Thanks to the growing power of social media, a landmark peer-reviewed paper (Lennerz et.al 2018) was published in the Journal of Pediatrics.[75] Though on the beginning wrung of evidence, the results are clear and evident and CAN NO LONGER BE IGNORED. It is NOT something that just works for me. And, it doesn't just improve control, it actually allows for normal blood glucose nearly around the clock. This promising new gold standard emerges in medical literature.

Prior to this publication, social media had allowed those of us using this method to connect and share experiences and provide needed support. I am in several groups: one using this for T1 kids, several for T2, and still others yet using this or vastly popular ketogenic diet for metabolic health and/or weight loss. We all held several things in common:

1. Dramatic improvement across metrics for metabolic health.
2. Astonishment at the simplicity of the remedy.
3. Utter shock at the lack of medical acceptance.
4. Dismay at the amount of grief and heartache we must all lay witness to as we watch others less fortunate than ourselves suffer at the hands of this terrible disease.

People react differently to the same situation. I watch this new, growing demographic of literally tens of thousands of people and I see the need to put their lives in context with this dichotomous situation. Like myself, many people, focus their efforts on trying to help people realize there is a better way. Unfortunately, the lack of medical knowledge and understanding of the safety and efficacy of carbohydrate restriction for diabetes and metabolic management blocks this work despite an undisputed critical review paper,[76] Feinman et al, published in 2015. https://www.researchgate.net/publication/263968313_Dietary_Car bohydrate_restriction_as_the_first_approach_in_diabetes_manage ment_Critical_review_and_evidence_base

Unfortunately, what I see most is an innate need to place blame. It is a literal rainbow of blame: the sugar industry for high fructose corn syrup, the fast food industry for trans-fats, the larger food industry for keeping us surrounded by food and food images, Big Pharma from profiting off of our misery, the ADA for lying to us while taking money from the food industry, the medical community for not protecting us and, finally, nutrition research for continuing to turn a blind eye to the growing body of evidence and misleading the public with confusing, poorly done epidemiologic research. This blame takes a myriad of forms and carries with it great passion and growing anger.

As a card-carrying health care professional observing this spectrum of outrage, I prefer to remain neutral and see the larger process from the advent of insulin through the attempts to understand heart disease and the current state that has come from the honest efforts to understand this large societal problem. I prefer to refrain from blame and engage in activities that seek to bring together the public, health care professionals and researchers.

However, I have had to personally watch my daughter go through adolescence and early adulthood trying to manage her diabetes amidst the public sea of nutritional misinformation. I see health care professionals whose hands are tied by well-worn clinical guidelines. In addition, I lay witness to the suffering of the masses at the hands of diabetes and the wasted healthcare dollars from the sequelae of the disease. And, I carry the prophetic burden of knowing that there is a better way. I feel responsible for those less fortunate than I, either financially or educationally, that have no voice. My patience is waning.

When I read the strategic plan, both sadness and disbelief overwhelm me. Why are the above evidence and more recent impressive evidence from Virta health (Halberg, et al 2018 published in Diabetes Therapy)[77] still ignored?

Why are the dietary patterns of Mediterranean and vegetarian diets still the mainstay of this plan despite lackluster evidence? How much money has the NIH already devoted in these outdated dietary strategies? Where are the results from this investment of OUR money? I am no accountant so please help me understand your continued backing of these strategies. I can only understand head to head clinical trials with these strategies against carbohydrate restriction. And, there is an ominous omission of very low carbohydrate diets that are notably now being studied by the USDA.

In a spirit of transparency, please provide a breakdown of money spent to study carbohydrate restriction compared to the money spent in the attempt to back the status quo, which has already proved only to exacerbate the metabolic problem in the US. If you really have a goal to target disease and disease prevention, you ignore the growing body of evidence for carbohydrate restriction at your own peril. The NIH will open itself up a wave of blame and anger unable to be contained.

I, personally, will no longer be able to refrain from placing blame.

And, I, the mother, the person with T2 diabetes, the health care professional, "I speak for the trees."

Carole Friend.

Chapter 26: When the patient is you or part of you

"If the situation is getting worse, then the only logical explanation is that our understanding and treatment of type 2 diabetes is fundamentally flawed."
Dr. Jason Fung.

E at three to four slices of whole wheat bread, five spoons of rice, three shares of fruits and five shares of vegetables, no fat and a medium amount of protein every day. Take your fast-acting insulin shots on time, as prescribed, and walk half an hour a day. Please be aware Mr. Syed, if you are not following these instructions, you will not be able to control your blood sugar," this is what Syed hears every visit to his famous endocrinologist Dr. Hazem.

Dr. Hazem is considered the best endocrinologist in diabetes management in his city. Indeed, every diabetic in the town knows he has no substitute. Syed literally follows the advice with no deviation. Nevertheless, his blood sugar is all over the place. It always fluctuates between 300 and 50 mg/dl and he really doesn't know why. Every time Syed shows his numbers to Dr. Hazem, he senses a blaming look and has to suffer some embarrassing comments about not following the sacred instructions!

Syed is a fifty-eight-year-old poor Egyptian man with a low-level education. He is working as a factory laborer all his life. He was diagnosed with T2 diabetes about 13 years ago and since then his health was deteriorating.

Health insurance for people like Syed is a privilege he cannot afford. He had to visit Dr. Hazem's clinic every three months and pay a fee of 300 Egyptian pounds from his pocket. The fee represents almost 20% of his tiny salary. Only 10 mins are allowed for Syed to sit with Dr. Hazem. The first five minutes, Syed listens to the same repeated advice and in the remaining five minutes, Syed always tries to get an answer for the sole question that has haunted his mind since he started seeing Dr. Hazem. He always tries to be cautious, when asking, not to press on Dr. Hazem's ego and not to show a challenging tone.

"Why are my BS numbers bad even though I exactly follow your instructions?" Syed asked carefully, trying not to look as he criticizes Dr. Hazem. He knows that such a question could provoke Dr. Hazem's anger.

Despite Syed's attempts to be cautious in asking, it was not well accepted by Dr. Hazem who felt intellectually intimidated by the question. He got red and angry. "You better off sitting on my seat, Mr. Syed! The internet has ruined your brain! It has made you guys think you are all doctors," Hazem said angrily.

At that moment, Syed realized he had to leave before it gets worse.

Moving forward, Syed's sight worsened, his feet became numb, and his kidney function deteriorated. Things were getting worse month after month. Three weeks after his last visit to Dr. Hazem's clinic, Syed was advised by a friend to take part in many low carbohydrate groups on the internet. Many of these groups have great credibility and have physician members who believe in this approach to managing diabetes.

After learning many things on those groups, Syed was filled with anger and decided to go and face Hazem with what he learned. Why wasn't he taught this way to control his BS? He went directly to the clinic with no prior reservation. He paid a higher fee to see Dr. Hazem on an urgent basis. The nurse took Syed to Hazem's office. Syed entered and immediately asked Hazem with an anxious and brittle voice: "I have almost gotten all the complications I was working hard to avoid in spite of doing what you advised exactly, so where was the problem, Dr. Hazem?"

"This is diabetes Mr. Syed–It is a progressive disease," Hazem said!

"During the last three weeks, I figured out that you were advising me to eat sugar for a long time. Why did you advise me to eat sugar if my body cannot handle sugar?" Syed said.

"What is this hallucination, Mr. Syed? I never advised you to eat sugar. Are you crazy?" Hazem said.

"Yes, you did doctor! I recently learned that whole-wheat bread you advised me to eat, for five years, contains Amylopectin-A, which is a starch that turns to glucose faster than sugar itself. You also advised me to eat rice, which every tablespoon has 5 to 7 grams of fast-acting carbohydrates that turns rapidly to glucose in my body! Moreover, every apple has about 20 grams of carbohydrate, which is about 5 spoons of sugar between glucose and fructose in it along with a little fiber! All these foods insanely raise my blood sugar day and night!" Syed said.

"This is bull sh.. Syed and I will not allow you to interfere in my work like that," Hazem said.

With an unstoppable agitated voice, "But I cut all starches including bread, rice, pasta, and potatoes to test this bull sh.. And, GUESS WHAT prof. Hazem! It was the first time in my whole life, as a diabetic, my blood sugar was between 80 to 100 mg/dl for a whole two weeks!" In addition, "I reduced my daily dose of fast-acting insulin by almost 60%." Syed said.

"This is an illusion Syed, your Facebook information will not be more credible than the international medical guidelines," Hazem said!

"I do not care about the guidelines anymore; I only care about my BS numbers. I had followed what you advised me for 5 years and all I got was a bad control and many complications. Now, with just simple changes on my diet, I have achieved the numbers I was dreaming of! I just wanted to share these results with you, so you could help other people with diabetes, in your clinic, getting the same fine results as well." Syed said.

"Well this is enough, you don't need me anymore. You are an expert now and nothing will make me happier than you step out of my office right now. Go ahead and look for another doctor or you know what, be your own doctor, Mr. Syed! Bye now." Hazem said, with an ironic accent.

Syed was shocked and boiling. He looked at Hazem straight in the eyes and said, "You do not even want to listen, read or research about what I told you. You only care about the guidelines. You don't care about the wellness of your patients. Before I leave, I just want to remind you that when you graduated, you swore not to harm patients, do you remember?"

While heading out of his office, Syed said, "If you are arguing out of ego and pride then you will regret this one day. I ask God to enlighten your insight, Dr. Hazem. Have a good night."

"You too... Have a good night," Hazem responded aggressively.

Deep in his heart, Hazem felt indescribable bitterness. He is a kind man by nature but he is going by the rulebook. As a physician, he must follow the guidelines he had been taught. He cannot be driven by internet practices. Certainly, he is extremely confident that what he advises his patients is matching with what he had learned. His conscience is content.

"So, why did such a simple semi-educated person like Syed hurt your conscience like that? How did he dare to accuse you of not caring about the wellness of your patients? That was extremely rude of him." Inner voice said.

His inner voice kept on telling him, "What is wrong with you Hazem, isn't your ultimate target is to achieve excellent BS numbers with your patients, so they could protect themselves against the deadly complications? What exactly upset you from Syed? Didn't you really swear not to cause harm to your patients as Syed said?" The inner voice said.

"Yes, I did!" Hazem replied.

What was the last book you read about diabetes management since you graduated Hazem? Twenty years ago, isn't it? The inner voice asked.

"Yes, true, about twenty years ago. Anyway, I have no more time to waste. I follow the guidelines and I believe I am doing the right thing." Hazem replied.

"Ok, fine. Stay calm and go on with your life," the inner voice said.

Hazem presses the ring to the nurse to let the next patient in.

After six months

The sixth-grade teacher was writing something on the board while students behind him were listening. The teacher heard a low voice saying, "I am too tired, I feel I will faint," and then he heard a sound of a body hit the ground. The teacher rushed to find out that student Ahmed Hazem fainted and fell on the floor. Ahmed was immediately taken to the hospital where his father was called in.

Dr. Hazem rushed to the hospital to find his son in a diabetic coma with a blood sugar of 860 mg/dl. Everyone in the hospital knows the famous endocrinologist, Dr. Hazem. He could barely stand on his feet at one of the room's corners with a devastated look and teary eyes.

A week later, Ahmed was discharged from the hospital and Dr. Hazem started dealing with his T1 diabetes, as he knew best. He took three weeks off his work to be with Ahmed in an attempt to control his blood sugar. He took care of the food, insulin, blood sugar monitoring. Unfortunately, Ahmed's blood sugar was either high or low despite Hazem's great experience in this field.

Hazem tried every way he knows, as an experienced endo, to normalize Ahmed's blood sugar but he could not do it at all. Only now, he started thinking of reading and exploring what he could really do to protect his own son from this killer.

"OMG, wait a minute," the inner voice knocked!

"I tried with Ahmed all the tricks I know and I followed all the advice I asked my diabetic patients to follow but I was not able to control his blood sugar. The whole wheat, the fruits, the vegetables, the ratios, the right amount of insulin according to age and weight, etc. Nevertheless, I failed." Inner voice said.

"I blamed many people who came to my clinic with high numbers and accused them of not being strict following my advice. And, here I am, figuring out that my advice was totally wrong. I always labeled them as weak and lacked will power! I defended the guidelines over anything else. I can see clearly now that those poor diabetics, my patients, were honest and just saying the truth. They were right and I was wrong. Shame on me that I only believe them now because the patient is my son!" inner voice said.

Hazem was filled with guilt. He left home, drove to his clinic at 10 pm, and started reading and searching like crazy. Again, his inner voice jumped in saying "Now only you research and read when the patient is your son! Why has not one of those suffering patients moved your desire to learn more to ease their pain, why?"

All of a sudden, the way he treated Syed jumped to his mind. He grasped the phone immediately and called him.

"Hi Syed, how are you? Can you please come over to my office immediately? Or else I can even come over to you. I just want to see you urgently," Hazem said.

"Any problem Dr. Hazem, your voice is not OK?" Syed said.

"I am fine Syed. I just want to see you please," Hazem said.

"Ok Dr. Hazem, just give me 30 minutes and I will be there," Syed said.

Syed arrived and Dr. Hazem was waiting for him in front of the building with an emotional hug saying, "Please accept my apology Syed, I am so sorry. You were right and I was wrong. Please forgive me."

"You worried me a lot this way. What happened?" Syed asked.

My son Ahmed was diagnosed with T1 diabetes and I really do not know how to control his blood sugar. I need your practical experience to achieve this, please!

Final Note

I never lost the sight of the big image while writing every chapter of this book. Every word leads to the same big goal of living with normal blood sugar. It is an unpleasant life, full of depression and pain, to live the sequelae of uncontrolled diabetes. Who wants to live a life with pain? Diabetes is not a death sentence as many of us think. It is a condition that can be dealt with, efficiently, if we want to. Controlling diabetes is a decision that cannot be postponed anymore. If the medical community has failed us (PWD), then we have to rise and defend our right to live with normal blood sugar. We definitely deserve that.

There are many methods out there lead to mediocre control of diabetes. But, in this book, I am only concerned about the real diabetes control, not the one defined by big organizations. As I said, my goal was never to force or preach my own understanding. Instead, my goal was to share what works well for many others and myself. I tried all other methods, one by one, but it did not work out to get the monster under control. You too, do not take my word for granted. In fact, I invite you to try every method; you might read or heard about. But, please do not let diabetes drags you until you face the undesired consequences. While trying, please be honest with yourself in judging what really brings good results and what don't. If you measure 160 mg/dl after food, do not believe any physician or organization who tells you that this number is a normal blood sugar number. It is your own health, not anyone else.

If you are a diabetic with complications, start immediately to normalize your blood sugar. That, itself, will reverse many complications and stop the deterioration of others. If you are new diagnosed diabetic or pre-diabetic, aim for the control as soon as you can, so you could reverse it. I know many newly diagnosed and pre-diabetics who were able to reverse their conditions just by committing to the right dietary choice, intermittent fasting, losing weight and exercise. It is not a miracle; it is just a process that needed be followed strictly and respectfully.

To be frank, I never blindly followed the low carb WOE. Not at all. I tried, experimented and monitored my blood sugar with or without low carb. I let the results decide which method I should follow. And the winner was the low carb. It doesn't have to be high fat or high protein. This is something left to you to decide. However, it has to be low carb in order for me to control my BS. Admittedly, no matter what I did to maneuver around the low carb, my blood sugar numbers repeatedly showed me I was wrong.

By the end of this book, I invite you to learn deeper about diabetes management, your nutritional needs, your medication, and your tools. I invite you to learn as Hamza did and to be Robert in supporting fellow diabetics. I urge you to find a doctor like Hazem after he recognized the truth and to be Suzan in taking care of your T1 child blood sugar. Please do not settle down for ordinariness when it comes to diabetes.

I pray that my message reach your heart and I hope that this book brought you a lasting benefit on the path of living a better life with diabetes.

Ahmed Afifi.

About The Author

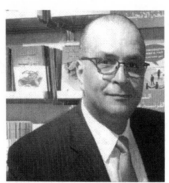

Ahmed Afifi, completed B.Sc. in Mechanical Power Engineering from The Alexandria University, Alexandra, Egypt. Ahmed is an insulin-dependent diabetic and an Associate diabetes educator accredited from AADE (American Association of Diabetes Educators). He was able to control his blood sugar after stumbling on Dr. Bernstein's book, <u>Dr. Bernstein's Diabetes Solution</u>. With proper management, Ahmed's HbA1c came down from 10% to 5.5%, his triglycerides were reduced from 1200 to 99 mg/dl.

Ahmed is an advocate for low carb WOE and is the author of two books written in Arabic, <u>What You Do Not Know About Diabetes</u> and <u>In Love, Life and Open Buffet</u>. He is so passionate about spreading the word about blood sugar control. He writes about health and diabetes management on his website and his Facebook page that has 22000 followers.

Having the experience of insulin-dependent diabetic with great numbers and diabetes education have allowed Ahmed to reach and support many diabetics all over the world. You can contact Ahmed through his email or his social network channels.

Website: www.ahmedafifi.net

Facebook: https://www.facebook.com/amdiabetic/

Twitter: https://twitter.com/afifi30

You Tube: https://bit.ly/2TNrh9g

Email: afifi30@gmail.com

Table of Abbreviations

AACE : American Association of Clinical Endocrinologists
ADA : American Diabetes Association
AGEs : advanced glycated end-products
AHPRA : The Australian Health Practitioners Regulatory Authority
BS : blood sugar
CF : correction factor
CHD : coronary heart disease
CHL : cholesterol
DKA : diabetes ketoacidosis
DP : dawn phenomenon
FAC : fast acting carbohydrates
FAI : fast acting insulin
FBT : fasting blood sugar test
HbA1c : Hemoglobin A1c test
HDL : high density lipoprotein
HFCS : high fructose corn syrup
HGH : Human growth hormone
HPCSA : the Health Professional Council of South Africa
HSL : High Sensitive Lipase
IC ratio : insulin to carbohydrate ratio
IDF : international diabetes federation
IOB : Insulin on Board
LADA : Latent Autoimmune Diabetes of Adults
LC : low carbohydrate
LCHF : Low Carb/High Fat diet
LDL : low density lipoprotein
LPL : Lipoprotein lipase
MDI : multi daily injections
MODY : mature onset diabetes of the young

Ahmed Afifi

MS : metabolic syndrome
OBS : Open Buffet Syndrome
PWD : people with diabetes
SN : sulfonylureas
T1: type one diabetes
T2 : type two diabetes
TDD : total daily insulin dos
TG : triglycerides
WHO : World Health Organization
WOE : way of eating

Index

D

E

F

Endnotes

[1] Rosengren, A., Jing, X., Eliasson, L., & Renström, E. (n.d.). Why Treatment Fails in Type 2 Diabetes. Retrieved from https://journals.plos.org/plosmedicine/article?id=10.1371/journal.pmed.0050215

[2] Bernstein, R. K. (2007). *Dr. Bernstein's diabetes solution: The complete guide to achieving normal blood sugars*. New York: Little, Brown and Company, p. 236.

[3] Bernstein, R. K. (2007). *Dr. Bernstein's diabetes solution: The complete guide to achieving normal blood sugars*. New York: Little, Brown and Company, p. 235.

[4] Diabetes. (2018, October 30). Retrieved from https://www.who.int/en/news-room/fact-sheets/detail/diabetes

[5] IDF diabetes atlas - 8th edition. (n.d.). Retrieved from http://diabetesatlas.org/resources/2017-atlas.html

[6] IDF diabetes atlas - 8th edition. (n.d.). Retrieved from http://diabetesatlas.org/resources/2017-atlas.html

[7] IDF diabetes atlas - 8th edition. (n.d.). Retrieved from http://diabetesatlas.org/resources/2017-atlas.html

[8] Luca. (2018, August 07). 10 Best Selling Drugs 2018 - Diabetes. Retrieved from https://www.igeahub.com/2018/08/07/10-best-selling-drugs-2018-diabetes/

[9] Bernstein, R. K. (207). *Dr. Bernstein's diabetes solution: The complete guide to achieving normal blood sugars*. New York: Little, Brown and Company.

[10] Diabetes. (2018, October 30). Retrieved from https://www.who.int/en/news-room/fact-sheets/detail/diabetes

[11] NDEI.org. (n.d.). Retrieved from http://www.ndei.org/ADA-diabetes-management-guidelines-glycemic-targets-A1C-PG.aspx.html

[12] Perlmutter, D., Loberg, K., & Ganim, P. (2013). *Grain brain the surprising truth about wheat, carbs, and sugar--your brains silent killers*. New York, NY: Hachette book group. pp. 65, 66.

[13] Moonishaa TM, Nanda SK, Shamraj M, Sivaa R, Sivakumar P, Ravichandran K. Evaluation of leptin as a marker of insulin resistance in type 2 diabetes mellitus. Int J App Basic Med Res [serial online] 2017 [cited 2019 Jan 17];7:176-80. Available from: http://www.ijabmr.org/text.asp?2017/7/3/176/212959

[14] Fung, J., & Moore, J. (2016). *The complete guide to fasting: Heal your body through intermittent, alternate-day, and extended fasting*. Las Vegas: Victory Belt Publishing. p. 168.

[15] Role of leptin resistance in the development of obesity in ... (n.d.). Retrieved from https://www.ncbi.nlm.nih.gov/pmc/articles/PMC3706252/

[16] Why is it so Hard to Maintain a Reduced Body Weight? (2011, May 18). Retrieved from http://www.drsharma.ca/obesitywhy-is-it-so-hard-to-maintain-a-reduced-body-weight

[17] Fung, J., & Moore, J. (2016). *The complete guide to fasting: Heal your body through intermittent, alternate-day, and extended fasting*. Las Vegas: Victory Belt Publishing, p. 49.

[18] How fasting affects your physiology and hormones. (2018, September 14). Retrieved from https://www.dietdoctor.com/fasting-affects-physiology-hormones

[19] Fung, J., & Moore, J. (2016). *The complete guide to fasting: Heal your body through intermittent, alternate-day, and extended fasting*. Las Vegas: Victory Belt Publishing.

[20] Fung, J., & Moore, J. (2016). *The complete guide to fasting: Heal your body through intermittent, alternate-day, and extended fasting*. Las Vegas: Victory Belt Publishing, p. 77.

[21] Fung, J., & Moore, J. (2016). *The complete guide to fasting: Heal your body through intermittent, alternate-day, and extended fasting*. Las Vegas: Victory Belt Publishing, p. 52.

[22] Fung, J., & Moore, J. (2016). *The complete guide to fasting: Heal your body through intermittent, alternate-day, and extended fasting*. Las Vegas: Victory Belt Publishing, p. 52.

[23] Hartman, M. L., Veldhuis, J. D., Johnson, M. L., Lee, M. M., Alberti, K. G., Samojlik, E., & Thorner, M. O. (1992, April). Augmented growth hormone (GH) secretory burst frequency and amplitude mediate enhanced GH secretion

during a two-day fast in normal men. Retrieved from
https://www.ncbi.nlm.nih.gov/pubmed/1548337

24 Catenacci, V. A., Pan, Z., Ostendorf, D., Brannon, S., Gozansky, W. S., Mattson, M. P., Donahoo, W. T. (2016, August 29). A randomized pilot study comparing zero-calorie alternate-day fasting to daily caloric restriction in adults with obesity. Retrieved from
https://onlinelibrary.wiley.com/doi/full/10.1002/oby.21581

25 Gotthardt, L., J., Yeomans, Yang, A., J., Yasrebi, . . . T., N. (2016, February 01). Intermittent Fasting Promotes Fat Loss With Lean Mass Retention, Increased Hypothalamic Norepinephrine Content, and Increased Neuropeptide Y Gene Expression in Diet-Induced Obese Male Mice. Retrieved from https://academic.oup.com/endo/article/157/2/679/2422759

26 Intermittent Fasting of High-Fat Diet Increases Hypothalamic Norepinephrine and Improves Metabolic Parameters in Obese Mice. (n.d.). Retrieved from http://www.fasebj.org/content/29/1_Supplement/LB231.short

27 Ruhl, J. (2016). *Blood sugar 101: What they don't tell you about diabetes*. Turners Falls, MA: Technion Books. Chapter 3. P, 17.

28 Overweight & Obesity Statistics. (2017, August 01). Retrieved from https://www.niddk.nih.gov/health-information/health-statistics/overweight-obesity

29 Type 2 diabetes mellitus in children and adolescent: An ... (2018, September 28). Retrieved from http://e-apem.org/upload/pdf/apem-2018-23-3-119.pdf

30 Davis, W. (2015). *Wheat belly: Lose the wheat, lose the weight and find your path back to health*. London: Harper Thorsons, p. 60.

31 Features of a successful therapeutic fast of 382 days ... (1973, March). Retrieved from https://www.ncbi.nlm.nih.gov/pmc/articles/PMC2495396/

32 Bernstein, R. K. (2011). *Dr. Bernsteins diabetes solution: The complete guide to achieving normal blood sugars*. New York: Little, Brown and Company, p, xvi.

33 What Is a Normal Blood Sugar. (n.d.). Retrieved from https://www.bloodsugar101.com/what-is-a-normal-blood-sugar

34 Ruhl, J. (2016). *Blood sugar 101: What they don't tell you about diabetes*. Turners Falls, MA: Technion Books. Chapter 1. P, 7.

35 Hunter, K. F., RN, MN, GNC (C), & More, K. N., RN, PhD. (n.d.). Retrieved from https://www.medscape.com/viewarticle/458587_3

36 Correction Factor. (2012, November 29). Retrieved from https://www.diabetesnet.com/diabetes-control/rules-control/correction-factor

[37] Correction Factor. (2012, November 29). Retrieved from https://www.diabetesnet.com/diabetes-control/rules-control/correction-factor

[38] Taubes, G. (2011). *Why we get fat: And what we can do about it*. New York: Anchor Books, p. 189, 190.

[39] Fung, J. (2016). *The Obesity Code: Unlocking the Secrets of Weight Loss*. Vancouver: Greystone Books.

[40] Emmerich, M. (2013). *Keto-adapted: Your guide to accelerated weight loss and healthy healing*, p. 30.

[41] Rodríguez-Morán, M., & Guerrero-Romero, F. (2003, April 01). Oral Magnesium Supplementation Improves Insulin Sensitivity and Metabolic Control in Type 2 Diabetic Subjects. Retrieved from http://care.diabetesjournals.org/content/26/4/1147

[42] Spero, D., & BSN. (2012, April 25). Magnesium: The Forgotten Healer. Retrieved from https://www.diabetesselfmanagement.com/blog/magnesium-the-forgotten-healer/

[43] Dean, C., & Dean, C. (2017). *The magnesium miracle*. New York: Ballantine Books.

[44] Emmerich, M. (2013). *Keto-adapted: Your guide to accelerated weight loss and healthy healing*, p. 31.

[45] Vitamin D deficiency linked to greater risk of diabetes. (2018, April 19). Retrieved from https://www.sciencedaily.com/releases/2018/04/180419154632.htm

[46] Park, K., Garland, C. F., Gorham, E. D., BuDoff, L., & Barrett-Connor, E. (n.d.). Plasma 25-hydroxyvitamin D concentration and risk of type 2 diabetes and pre-diabetes: 12-year cohort study. Retrieved from http://journals.plos.org/plosone/article?id=10.1371/journal.pone.0193070

[47] Vitamin D - Proven to Help Prevent Breast Cancer. (2014, March 13). Retrieved from http://ubcf.org/vitamin-d-proven-to-help-prevent-breast-cancer/

[48] Emmerich, M. (2013). *Keto-adapted: Your guide to accelerated weight loss and healthy healing*, p. 175.

[49] Saul, A. W. (n.d.). Retrieved from http://www.doctoryourself.com/vitaminc.html

[50] Ruhl, J. (2016). *Blood sugar 101: What they don't tell you about diabetes*. Turners Falls, MA: Technion Books, p, 5.

[51] Piemonte, L. (2018, November 19). Hypoglycaemia. Retrieved January 11, 2019, from https://idf.org/52-about-diabetes.html

[52] Lennerz, B. S., Barton, A., Bernstein, R. K., Dikeman, R. D., Diulus, C., Hallberg, S., . . . Ludwig, D. S. (2018, June 01). Management of Type 1 Diabetes With a Very Low–Carbohydrate Diet. Retrieved from http://pediatrics.aappublications.org/content/141/6/e20173349

[53] https://optimisingnutrition.com/2016/02/22/optimising-blood-sugars-with-rd-dikeman/

[54] 42 (Supplement 1). (2019, January 01). Retrieved from http://care.diabetesjournals.org/content/42/Supplement_1

[55] Fung, J. (2016). *The Obesity Code: Unlocking the Secrets of Weight Loss.* Vancouver: Greystone Books.

[56] Taubes, G. (2011). *Why we get fat: And what we can do about it.* New York: Anchor Books. Pp, 119, 120.

[57] Taubes, G. (2011). *Why we get fat: And what we can do about it.* New York: Anchor Books, pp. 127, 128.

[58] Perlmutter, D., Loberg, K., & Ganim, P. (2013). *Grain brain the surprising truth about wheat, carbs, and sugar--your brains silent killers.* New York, NY: Hachette book group

[59] https://www.medicines.org.uk/emc/files/pil.6585.pdf

[60] Davis, W. (2015). *Wheat belly: Lose the wheat, lose the weight and find your path back to health.* London: Harper Thorsons, pp, 106, 107.

[61] Bernstein, R. K. (2011). *Dr. Bernsteins diabetes solution: The complete guide to achieving normal blood sugars.* New York: Little, Brown and Company, p. 103.

[62] Bernstein, R. K. (2011). *Dr. Bernsteins diabetes solution: The complete guide to achieving normal blood sugars.* New York: Little, Brown and Company, p. 103

[63] Bernstein, R. K. (2011). *Dr. Bernsteins diabetes solution: The complete guide to achieving normal blood sugars.* New York: Little, Brown and Company, pp. 105, 106.

[64] Bernstein, R. K. (2011). *Dr. Bernstein's diabetes solution: The complete guide to achieving normal blood sugars.* New York: Little, Brown and Company, p, 105.

[65] Bernstein, R. K. (2011). *Dr. Bernstein's diabetes solution: The complete guide to achieving normal blood sugars.* New York: Little, Brown and Company, p, 102.

[66] https://www.youtube.com/watch?v=faJtPTMQIU4

[67] Yajun Liang, Davide Liborio Vetrano, & Chengxuan Qiu. (2017, December 28). Serum total cholesterol and risk of cardiovascular and non-cardiovascular mortality in old age: A population-based study. Retrieved from https://bmcgeriatr.biomedcentral.com/articles/10.1186/s12877-017-0685-z

[68] Does Accumulation of Advanced Glycation End Products ... (n.d.). Retrieved from https://www.ncbi.nlm.nih.gov/pmc/articles/PMC2920582/

[69] Perlmutter, D., Loberg, K., & Ganim, P. (2013). *Grain brain the surprising truth about wheat, carbs, and sugar--your brains silent killers*. New York, NY: Hachette book group. P, 38.

[70] Superko, H. R. (n.d.). Small, dense, low-density lipoprotein and atherosclerosis. Retrieved from https://link.springer.com/article/10.1007/s11883-000-0024-1

[71] Emmerich, M. (2013). *Keto-adapted: Your guide to accelerated weight loss and healthy healing*, p. 47.

[72] Nordestgaard, B. G., Benn, M., Schnohr, P., & Tybjærg-Hansen, A. (2007). Nonfasting Triglycerides and Risk of Myocardial Infarction, Ischemic Heart Disease, and Death in Men and Women. *Jama,298*(3), 299. doi:10.1001/jama.298.3.299.

[73] Cholesterol-reducing Drugs May Lessen Brain Function, Says Researcher. (2009, February 26). Retrieved from https://www.sciencedaily.com/releases/2009/02/090223221430.htm

[74] Jenny. (2012, October 31). New Page: Why Lowering HbA1c Below 6.0% Is Not Dangerous. Retrieved from https://phlauntdiabetesupdates.blogspot.com/2012/10/new-page-why-lowering-a1c-below-60-is.html

[75] Lennerz, B. S., Barton, A., Bernstein, R. K., Dikeman, R. D., Diulus, C., Hallberg, S., . . . Ludwig, D. S. (2018, June 01). Management of Type 1 Diabetes With a Very Low–Carbohydrate Diet. Retrieved from http://pediatrics.aappublications.org/content/141/6/e20173349

[76] Dietary Carbohydrate restriction as the first approach in ... (2014, September). Retrieved from https://www.researchgate.net/publication/263968313_Dietary_Carbohydrate_restriction_as_the_first_approach_in_diabetes_management_Critical_review_and_evidence_base

[77] Effectiveness and Safety of a Novel Care Model for the ... (2018, April). Retrieved from https://link.springer.com/content/pdf/10.1007/s13300-018-0373-9.pdf